Conflict and Connection:
Anatomy of Mind and Emotion

Michael Jones MD

Contents:

Preface

This book can be best prefaced by seeing for yourself what this one exercise can tell you about the common sources of stress in your life.

Circle, or number in order of importance, what you feel are the three best attributes, and three least important attributes of these twenty-one:

Fairness
Forgiveness
Open-mindedness
Kindness
Enthusiasm
Compassion
Appreciation
Teamwork
Prudence
Curiosity
Love
Perseverance
Acceptance
Hope
Leadership
Humility
Creativity
Social Intelligence
Honesty
Investigation
Humor

Now, circle, or number in order of importance, the three attributes you feel are the worst, the ones you avoid the most because they have no or few redeeming qualities to them. Also, circle or number in order the three least bad attributes or ones you see some redeeming quality in:

Exploitation (taking advantage)
Obligation (guilting)
Intolerance
Fake or Unkind
Rage
Provoking Pity (Being Pathetic)
Complaining
Leeching (free-loading)
Fanaticism (tribalism)
Pride
Bartering (loving with strings attached)
Relentlessness (bothersome)
Competitiveness
Skepticism
Manipulation
Intrusiveness(nosey)
Uncreativity (plagiarism)
Exclusion(cliquey)
Deceit
Ego inflation
Dogmatization (ideological thinking)

Realizing bias in perception of what, because of our experience, catches and takes hold of our attention more than everything else, increases our perception and possible actions because we will know there is more to look for than we immediately see. Taking just a few seconds to consider whether there is more to a situation than what is at play on the top of our list of twenty-one interpersonal weapons, we might see something that offsets or outweighs it. The goal is to see things as they really are, so that we can interact with the actual thing and not our imagination of it. Our imagination of the line between interpersonal tools and weapons can be so biased that what we rank as the top three worst and top three least bad on the list can be completely opposite as someone else.

Whether we consciously think about it or not, we have lines already drawn because of our experience between what is positive and negative, and use that line to determine our actions. For example, there is a line between being aggressive, and being assertive. If our past experience tells us that aggression is really dangerous, we are more likely to include more things than we should in our definition of what qualifies as aggression. This will lead to that definition encroaching on what we define as being assertive. This can happen to the point where almost all assertiveness is considered aggressive, even merely stating our opinion.

The goal of this portion of the book, is to find those interpersonal weapons which in our mind have a definition broader than it should be, and then establishing the line between it and the actual definition of the corresponding interpersonal tool. The definition of an interpersonal weapon can expand to the point that both what actually is a weapon, and what actually is a tool, all are considered weapons... and therefore taboo. The opposite also happens, when our definitions of interpersonal tools are so big that they encroach on the definition of the interpersonal weapon—this leads to both what is actually a tool and what actually is a weapon, falsely all being considered tools.

The overall goal is to be able to recognize the right tool for the job and using it. The first step to figuring out what tool is right for the job is realizing that all the tools are equally good or productive when that is the right tool for the job. Likewise, all of the interpersonal weapons are equally bad, because anything but the right tool for a job is the wrong one. Which tool we use shouldn't be determined by which one we are familiar with, nor what using that tool might say about us to others. When our action is more based on what it might say about our identity than the nature of the action itself, we end up doing actions that are meaningless and counterproductive.

My intention of outlining someone of the logical implications of avoiding one taboo more than another is merely to seed the idea of the general form a bias could take—it is up to you to look into it further with past and present experiences. What you listed as the top three worst on the list of interpersonal tools is the common source of stress, and the three you listed as least bad are how that stress manifests.

Looking at past experiences should show a trend of what stresses you and how you react. That information can help you in the present catch yourself when you are reacting in what on the list you think is least bad and be able to check yourself to see if that is what you really want to do. Also, future situations can be better assessed for likely stressors, and you can decide before you go whether it will be worth it or plan how you will not let it derail you once you are there.

Logical Implications of strong taboos:

Exploitation: The Rescuer

We often end up doing much more than our share. We do this to the point that we tend to allow the impulse to look after the needs of someone else take precedence over the impulse to take care of our own needs.

Not only do we spend less time and energy on ourselves, but that little time we do spend is not as enjoyable or helpful because the distracting guilt we often feel while doing it.

We love helping people be successful, and we often do that by either protecting them from being taken advantage or by helping them protect themselves. We are very willing to take the time to explain things to people when they ask or need help, and we don't mind helping them learn at their own pace.

Obligation: The Hospitable

Because of how much we stress over making sure someone who is helping us feels appreciated, and how much effort we put into making sure they know they don't actually have to help, whatever someone is helping us with we could have probably just done ourselves would have been less stressful. We really don't like to bother other people, and so we end up just doing a lot of things by ourselves, even if in reality others would like to help if we asked

We don't enjoy the type of tension in relationships that comes from unspoken resentments or grudges. For this reason, we often try not to ask much of people or hold them to things they promise us.

As grateful as we are to receive gifts it still stresses us out because we don't want play the awkward game of seeing if they expect a gift in return and if so whether we can get them an equivalent gift that they don't think is better or worse than theirs.

Intolerance: The Humane

We like to give people a fair chance by giving them the benefit of the doubt and not hastily jump to conclusions that they have bad intent or a faulty plan.

We know that the things we do aren't perfect, we don't hold people to our idea of a perfect standard, and we don't want people holding us to their idea of a perfect standard either.

If we are going to err, we try to err on the side of being too accepting rather than err on the side of being too rejecting.

We prefer hanging out with friends one on one or in small groups because or friend groups can differ so much that it is hard at time to avoid tension.

We appreciate things that are hard to polarize, which is one reason why the outdoors is so appealing to us. We like getting away from places that are intellectual or emotional battlegrounds and out into the drama-free haven of nature.

Fake or Unkind: The Guardian Angel

We believe that kindness is contagious, and that a kind word, deed or even just a genuine smile is all it take sometimes to bring out the best in someone. We are vigilant about noticing sparks of good intent we can help turn into a flame.

We don't like fake compliments, and so we have become good at noticing and giving genuine ones. We love helping people be their best self.

We try to be excited when people are excited and sad when they are sad.

We look out for people so that we can know when someone needs help right when they need it.

Rage: The Peacemaker

Difficult situations run so much smoother when people remain calm instead of making them harder by losing their temper. Rage rarely if ever makes a situation better, and it's not hard to notice how much worse it gets when one person's rage sets off a chain reaction of other people losing their temper.

It's really hard for us to look up to someone who loses control to rage especially over small things despite whatever other accomplishments they have.

We don't lose our tempter, but it can be very irritating when someone or something prevents us from doing simple tasks the nice or polite way. Because of this we try to look ahead for things that might make things difficult in order to be ready to meet them calmly. We know that we don't think clearly when we are angry, and so we avoid doing things in the heat of the moment.

It is very frustrating if we slip up and take out frustration on someone, because we feel so passionately that it is wrong. Although, no matter how justified we feel getting mad at someone, we always end up getting mad at ourselves for doing it. This means that when we do vent our frustration on someone, we add the extra future frustration of being mad at ourselves to what someone already did to frustrate us.

Provoking pity: The Ascetic

Especially in situations where we feel others need courage to lean on, we often put on a good face and pretend that everything is great, even in dire circumstances.

If it feels like our life is falling apart and then attention gets brought to our situation, it only makes it more difficult for us—we don't want the situation compounded by rumors or by people treating us like we are sick or broken when really we are just tired or things are out of our control.

We rarely have time to enjoy the satisfaction of accomplishments because we are always pushing our limits into new territories and on to the next mountain to climb.

We don't get sympathy because we always look like we are handling life fine, and because we curtail the negative details when asked about stressful things. When someone is just being pathetic, it is very hard to sift through what they say for the real part of story.

We don't like sifting through any possible bay for attention in us, that we dismiss difficult or negative emotions.

Complaining: The Resilient

We typically avoid saying anything except positive things unless we make our complaint as factual and as least emotional as possible. If there is a confidant we can trust knows that we actually want to fix our problems and not just complain, we will tell the difficulty we are working with, and ask for suggestions on how to take action. Even with a confidant however, we are still careful not to appear that we don't want to take responsibility for our own problems. When we finally do tell someone about something difficult in our life, we make sure to include a plan and maybe even a timeline of accomplishing it. When a confidant is not available, we tend to isolate ourselves which often results in our condition slowly worsening.

We stay positive by doing nice things for other people. Since we spend more time working then complaining, we get a lot done and become proficient in whatever obstacle is in our way. With our large skill set, we are often asked for help. Sometimes when we hear others complain about something, we want to fix their problem for them just so that we don't have to hear them whining anymore.

Leeching: The Responsible

We rarely if ever leave a job half done. We don't need any help and definitely don't want anyone micromanaging us. Hopefully you are your own boss because no boss deserves you. We do more work than anyone on the team and need less oversight. We carry our own weight and more.

If we are at a social gathering, we feel significantly more comfortable if we can be working—we will find ourselves running the grill or washing dishes even if it's not our house. We are usually at get-togethers early to set up, there late to help clean up, and it is very possible that we never stopped working from start till finish... whether or not that was the plan. We are the ones most likely to randomly bring drinks or dessert to a party, which usually accounts for part of the reason we are invited to a number of events.

Fanaticism: The pragmatic

Especially in situations where people's opinions are emotionally charged, we often try to stay focused on things that most people can agree are essential to life or justifiable because of their connection to health, learning or something else unanimously considered beneficial.

We don't like when things are exaggerated. We don't believe in magic pills or cure-alls.

We care about people not the mask they wear. We don't see people as one idea that we either love or hate, but as many different ideas, some we agree with, and others we might not.

We know no one sees everything exactly the way we do, and we are okay with that—we appreciate uniqueness.

It's sad to us to see that some of the most authentic people or things we find don't always move forward only because whoever made them spent their time being awesome and didn't spend their time self-promoting. Because of that we like to fight against self-promoting and fighting for the underdog.

Pride: The Sage

We care more about what is being said than who is saying it, and what is being done more than who is doing it. We try to act and speak so that our words and deeds can stand on their own merit and not on someone's perception of us.

In group situations, we want everyone to be able to voice their opinion and have them considered, sometimes to the point of sacrificing making our opinion heard as much as we probably could or should.

We try not to feel entitled to special positions and treatment. It is difficult for us to write a resume because we don't like trying to make ourselves sound good on paper or quantify things that shouldn't be measure or bragged about, for example virtues or charity.

We love learning, but it's sad that learning makes us self-conscious sometimes.

Bartering: The Idealist

It's not that we are a hopeless romantic or in a fairytale world, we just aren't going to let social conventions or laziness keep us from really understanding love and loving the fullest possible. It is odd to us that people invest so much time in understanding some things that seem pretty unimportant to astounding depts but then take the surface-level understanding of love and don't seem to care to figure it out deeper. We can't understand how someone would argue to the point of being hurtful over what day of the week something occurred when telling a story. If we can't have a love deeper than that we would rather just not have love.

We like spontaneous adventures because in new situations people have to actually think to act instead of act out of habit. For this same reason we like to ask deep questions that really gets to the core of people. Because our conversations are intense, we get together with people sporadically instead of as a daily routine.

We avoid looks or feels like a business-like trading of services. We avoid putting conditions on what we give people. We don't like gifts when it is just seems like a formality. We are the ones most likely to give very random gifts or make very random gestures of love that are people find either very sincere and useful, or just think it odd.

Relentlessness: The Graceful

We are very conscientious, and dislike inconveniencing people. It doesn't matter if it is our birthday, we don't want others to think we require special treatment. If something doesn't happen naturally or without bothering anyone, we don't want to push it.

To avoid bothering people, we try to be attentive to what others say they like and dislike, and ask if we are not sure. We typically take at face-value what people say.

We notice when others start saying something and then stop. When that happens we try to get them to actually say or ask what they wanted to.

Competitiveness: The Quiet Confident
We have talents, but dislike becoming a target of competition or feeling pressured that to win or consistently win, we would have to stoop down to the level of our opponents and play dirty. It makes it not worth it to us. When people get competitive they cheat or get angry, and it easy ruins whatever activity, that didn't need any competitiveness to be fun anyway.

It's not that we don't see any value in competition, we like having a goal to work for and the motivation that comes by seeing someone do something awesome. Unless there is someone that we can compete with that we know plays fair and just likes the motivation, as soon as something we are doing starts to feel like a game, we try to get out of it.

Skepticism: The Optimist
We strongly dislike the idea of hastily dismissing an idea's potential just on face value. We know that if we focus on the negative first of an idea we might not be motivated to look into the positives and in the cases where the positives out weigh the negative, we wouldn't know.

We are not ones to say always or never when talking about something. We would rather have a definitive reason why we are or are not doing something rather than just having the vague feeling that it has always been good or bad for us.

Manipulation: The Confidant
Late night intimate conversations with people is very frequent occurrence for us despite not planning them. We like to know where someone is at emotionally, and work hard to help people feel safe expressing how they feel.

We try to be as forthcoming and transparent as possible with our plans and motives, that way people can make a clear decision whether they want to come along with us or not. If we invite someone else along with us, we feel overly responsible to make it a good experience—we can handle accidents that happen to ourselves but feel deeply responsible for them when they happen to others.

We sometimes have a hard time saying "no." This can lead to us getting walked over sometimes.

We try to be more supportive than critical, especially not giving too specific of advice. We want someone using their best judgment, not feeling like a failure and then just doing what other people say. We want someone to believe our advice because they see the value and logic in it, not because we broke their self-confidence or outsmarted them.

We likely enjoy using humor. We really want people to feel comfortable opening up, and we often use our sense of humor to do it.

Intrusiveness: The Philosopher

Our inner word is typically so rich and complex that is doesn't make sense to other people. It's not that we don't want to let people in, but our ideas are so interconnected that it is hard to find a place to start or a person willing to make the whole journey to understand. We would rather people make assumptions about our theories only in hindsight after they have seen them work, and not before when they can't comprehend why we are doing it.

We strongly dislike gossip and when others do around us we often try to change the topic or defend the person they are gossiping about.

We avoid asking questions that could be too personal. We are not scared to have personal conversations with others, but the setting has to be right and the feeling mutual.

Uncreativity: The Dreamer

Life is not black and white or flat to us, and that is because we look at things from every angle. We are not interested in following the crowd in an idea or action, We are focused on the idea or action itself and how we can improve it. We can tell we have figured out what something is when we can not only replicate it but make it better. We are not scared to try and fail, that is typically how we find out how to make something better is to see where it breaks. Most people don't share our same excitement for what there is to be found in trying new things and possibly failing.

Since every time something breaks we excitedly start thinking how we can improve it, and since things always break, especially because of how much we like testing things, we can get caught up in continually changing things.

We are self-motivated, and though we can be an asset in collaborating, often we work best when left alone. We don't work on a project linearly, because we want to consider as many possibilities as we can, we only narrow our focus when either ideas coalesce, or the deadline demands it.

Exclusion: The Social Architect

We spend a lot of time trying to understand people and situations well enough that we can peacefully integrate very different people into the same situation... people that otherwise probably wouldn't get along or care to try. This means that we can rarely relax and enjoy group situations, because we have to be busy predicting what people will do well enough to prevent the types of situations that will lead to drama or awkwardness.

We plan activities with a purpose, and usually have one or two people in mind for an event to help them. We want to help people be the person we know they can be, but sometimes the person we put the event on for ruins it by not being their best self despite so much effort to help create the situation where they can be.

What we notice first when entering a room is who is alone, and quickly focus on figuring out why they are alone and what we can do to include them. We value other people who help us in this effort. We know it often takes more effort and more time to include everyone, but that it's worth it.

Deceit: The Diplomat

We are as transparent and forthcoming as possible, even sometimes when it comes at the expense of negative repercussions that could have been avoided using discretion.

We likely feel that being misleading or withholding information is basically the same as lying. We don't like withholding important information from to thers and don't like people doing it to us.

We usually try to articulate our thoughts carefully in order to be as transparent as possible while at the same time not offending anyone... a task that is near impossible. Sometimes we get stressed when the process of articulating an answer that is transparent and forthcoming gets rushed.

We find that the best way to be honest and not offensive is to lay something out thoroughly so that it is all seen in context. It is very frustrating when we have rehearsed an extensive doctoral level dissertation to explain something that is a sensitive topic, and someone doesn't let us get it all out... then gets mad because only because they took it the wrong way. It is frustrating when someone summarizes what we said, not only overly simplifying it, but only focusing on certain parts and twisting them out of context. It is irritating when someone else feels like we offended them after we made a big effort not to.

We would rather tell the truth and accept the consequences, not only because we don't want a lie to come back and bite us later, but also because we don't want someone else to feel lied to.

Ego Inflation: The Valiant

Strength of character is more important to us than fame, power or money. We don't like how everything a person does reflects back on them depending on how it is perceived and that there is a pressure in society to do things in order to be seen and do other things we shouldn't and think its fine as long as we are not seen. We try to be the same person wherever we are and to do the right thing no matter what people will think of us for doing it.

We focus on pushing an idea forward and building on it rather than pushing forward our ego or building on it. We don't care for discussing people but would rather discuss things and best of all discuss ideas.

Dogmatization: The Scientist

We will listen to what people speak, but we won't believe until we test it for ourselves. We have a hard time jumping onboard with thinks that can't be tested especially if it seems convenient to someone that we can't test them. We may be involved in religion or politics, but if we do, each individual belief is clearly defined.

We don't like ideas that are convoluted. We like to take the time to deconstruct ideas presented to us so we know what to do with it.

Since we are not the type of people who jump into anything pre-emptively, when we do jump into something people notice. Once we finally get on board with something, hesitant people usually come along because they trust our judgement. This leads to people trying to convince us to endorse things because our opinion matters to other people—this can be annoying.

Considering the logical consequences of strong taboos for myself, I can definitely see which have affected my life the most. Some have remained consistent in my life, and others were stronger only for a time. I can't recall the exact inciting event or chain of events that lead to me strongly tabooing it, but uncreativity apparently has been something I have strongly avoided, and it has had quite the pronounced consequence on my life—my motivation to look outside of the box for the answers to understanding mind, emotion and connection is probably not a coincidence.

Something I was aware was very taboo to me, but didn't realize to what extent, was exclusion. I am not sure if this is because I came from a very inclusive family, or whether it was because I was sometimes excluded at school, or both, but the consequences of it in my day-to-day life are quite apparent. I have been to many parties and get-togethers where I was very stressed because I was trying to be the peace-keeper and help everyone feel included. It's probably also not a coincidence that I couldn't stop writing and rewriting until I found a way to present the answer of my question of mind and emotion in a way that was as accessible as possible to everyone, both in format and content.

The consequences of strong taboos are not always negative, that's one reason why we keep them. For example, it has been a good thing, trying to find a better way to explain to others what I discovered for myself, because that lead to discovering many more implications of what I found. It is actually a very complicated process to simplify and idea, that is probably the reason there is a saying, "you don't really know something until you can teach it."

Another benefit is that I have already had many people express the positive difference this book has made for them. There have been many good things, but they have come at a cost, a cost that is difficult to calculate because of my bias towards the interpersonal tools and weapons I happen to like and dislike. There's no way to say how my life would have been otherwise, and whether I would have felt as passionate about the book if the experiences that influenced my likes and dislikes had been different.

It is difficult to say whether our wounds go deeper than our convictions and what percentage that plays into our bias. I am neither promoting the nature nor the nurture theory of development, because either way we are left with a choice, to let our biology or circumstance determine our choices, or to choose for ourselves. I found it is possible to discover and start to eliminate bias whatever the cause may be.

Considering the influences of the taboos we hold verses the ideals, I think that often the taboos have more influence on our reflexes which means that the more stressed we get the more they can influence our actions. This is because though we would all like to be an ideal at something, entering a room, it is more likely that something we do will make us taboo, and less likely that we will meet an ideal. If we can't at least avoid looking bad, how could we expect to look good?

We likely come into a room and first look for potential dangers of things that could make us or label us as taboo. After considering those top three or so possible taboos, we then consider what to work towards in order to be ideal. Taboos likely get considered first when determining action, and potential actions are eliminated on the grounds of possibly being considered taboo, even if they had potential to be ideal. How many things have we wanted to do but didn't because we were scared it was taboo, and later wish we had?

We often abandon good ideas just because of the fear that we might fail at carrying them out. The fear of being taboo because of failure will confine us to only the things we think work because we have already done them or we have seen other people have done them and they seemed to work.

I didn't include a section of answers for what our top three favorite interpersonal tools imply, because the logical consequence of overusing a tool is in some ways a lot more obvious than overly avoiding specific taboos. Also, discovering all the potential consequence of overusing a tool will take a lifetime and is a personal journey we should all take. Even just describing the consequence of strong taboos fully would be a quite the task. I merely gave a short and haphazard synopsis of a few consequences each.

The overarching complication for holding strong taboos, is that when we don't have a clear definition for an interpersonal tool, the definition for the corresponding weapon can get too big and inclusive, or so small it doesn't apply to very many things. Saying "aggressiveness only means physically hurting people," would be an example of a definition way too small. Saying that "speaking your mind is almost always aggressive" is a definition that is way too big.

The point is not to take an interpersonal tool we use a lot and change it for one we are not familiar with. The point is to try to figure out when one of our favorite tools is the appropriate one, and when it's not—only the right tool for the right job will work, we can't just keep using our favorite tools for everything. In the long run nothing will make life easier than to figure out what tool to use and using it. A good definition of an interpersonal tool helps us understand exactly when to use it and when not to.

The list of interpersonal tools and weapons I derived, are from what I have outlined as the seven emotional lenses and the three systems of the psyche. These emotional lenses and systems of the psyche were the product primarily of my own experience, which I then compared to historical accounts of other people's experiences. I essentially did a cross-sectional study of the history of thought and emotion, from the Egyptian book of the dead written more than 3200 years ago which outlines seven parts of the soul, to today where facial expressions are distinguished by seven different emotions that neuroscience confirms are distinct circuits, and everything in between. My idea of the three systems of the psyche is illustrated well in Williams Foster's conclusion that all stories throughout history have one of three plots, 1) doing what feels right but seems illogical, 2) doing what seems logical but seems wrong, or 3) just repeating what was done before. There are many other concepts like, heart, mind and soul, Id, Ego and Super Ego, that all correlate pretty well with my theory.

I did not start this journey looking for a trick that merely would work to improve my life a little, but to really get to the bottom of things, and figure out how our mind and emotion is really wired. I figured that if I can't trust my perception of thoughts and feelings, and I can't trust what other people have written about their thoughts and feelings, that there would be no hope of ever finding the deepest answers to life.

In the journey to be able to trust my perception, I tried everything I could find to get rid of bias. The first bias, or indication of bias I found was emotionally charged language, which seemed to be everywhere, and was a cover for what someone is scared doesn't actually have value but wants it to have. I started reading books and articles and circling all the emotionally charged words. (By which I mean impossible words like "always, never, best ever, worst ever, etc.") I don't know why it didn't occur to me first, but eventually I realized that I could read my own journal and other things I have written, and I was embarrassed to see how much emotionally charged language there was in pretty much everything I wrote. I tried to edit what I wrote so it wouldn't be emotionally changed, by trying to find what I had really wanted to say but couldn't find the words for. I then tried to do the same for what other people wrote and hypothesize what the ideas and feelings they couldn't find words for were. Just that process alone changed my perception a lot, and seeing the change in my life by trying to avoid using emotionally charged language showed me a lot of things about life and about myself.

I found when I factoring in the assumption that our deepest drive was to love and be love, that editing out the emotionally charged language for the real thoughts and feelings was very straight forward. Often we look at language and try to analyze each word of a sentence from what we know about that word instead of analyzing each sentence for what it has to do with loving or being loved. We don't say or write things that don't make sense to us. It is more likely that someone is operating on a false assumption of what is means to love and be loved rather than that they are operating on something besides love. Looking in to all the false assumptions I somehow picked up about love, and knowing that some people have grown up in much more difficult situations than me, it makes sense that some people would have very false assumptions about love.

Though seeing the impact of emotionally charged language on my life helped a lot, instead of pacifying my desire to get to the bottom of things, it gave me hope that I really could do it—so I continued forward. I created a spreadsheet as I collected all the schools of thought I could find on the nature of mind and emotion. I started lining up what was common between them, and then began testing what was consistent between many or all the schools of thought. There was no specific answer I wanted to find, no point I was trying to prove, I had no idea when or even if what I had compiled would sort out into a concise answer or theory, but it did!

I tested it on myself and it worked. I started talking to other people about it, and quickly found a really strong correlation between ways that people approach situations now and their earliest memories—that was quite a shock!

In talking to someone I noticed they kept using the same few adjectives to describe different things, either for the positive or negative, which seemed odd because I knew they had a large vocabulary and were capable of using more specific words. Then after asking them about their earliest memories, I realized it probably wasn't a coincidence that those few favorite adjectives each person seemed to prefer directly had to do with their early memories. After quite a few people showed the same correlation, I knew there had to at least be something there. I correlated these adjectives to seven categories, which I call aspects of value, and tentatively associated them with the seven emotions, and that's when I realized I had really stumbled onto something important.

I was helping a friend quite smoking, and as I thought about it, I wondered which aspects of value smoking would seem positive, because I couldn't relate to wanting to smoke. Smoking, I determined, could be considered positive in two or three of the seven aspects of value, which were not the ones in my earliest memories. I asked my friend what her earliest memories where, and sure enough, the aspects of value most at play in her earliest memories were the two where smoking was positive. I told her this, and instead of trying to convince her of how I saw smoking, I went one-by-one through the aspects of value and asked her how she thought smoking applied. Considering each of the seven one-by-one she came to the same conclusion as I had. I realized then that we rarely give more than three reasons for something, and that our three reasons are usually in reference to the same three aspects of value. This would mean any time she considered quitting smoking before, the same three arguments would result in the same conclusion, that it was worth it to quit smoking.

It is easier to see both the good and the bad in others, and so each observation I made, I tried to apply to myself, and found that once I could see the general trend of something in someone else, not only could I start seeing it in myself, but I could take the investigation of it further. Then I would use what I found in myself to look for similarities in other people. I found that we all have three favorite aspects of value, and that we perceive life in reference to them. This eventually led to the survey. I explain the history of my discovery of it so that you know it is not a gimmick, and that hopefully it piques your interest enough to want to understand the foundational ideas that support the idea of the interpersonal tools and weapons I have outlined.

Introduction

We are born crying, not because we are hungry or out of pain, but just to be held. We are social creatures, to the extent that we will even opt to forego food or experience pain just to connect or stay connected with someone we care about. So why is connection so difficult? Why do we sometimes feel we are not enough to be loved? Why do we sometimes feel hopeless or broken?

We see things through emotional lenses which are tailored to assess unique aspects of value. One emotional lens is not enough to see and understand life, ourselves, or others. I propose there are seven aspects of value which match up with our seven emotions. Emotions are neither positive nor negative. Emotions are merely the conclusion of our intuition of the pivotal aspect of value in a situation and what general or fundamental approach to make.

The seven emotions and corresponding aspects of value are:

1) Contempt - functionality/purpose
2) Sadness - accuracy/reproducibility
3) Surprise - exploration/perspective
4) Happiness - response/continuity
5) Anger - stability/strength
6) Fear - protection/preservation
7) Disgust - excellence/transcendence.

It is possible to survive operating in life using only one emotional lens, but not to thrive—to thrive we must actually see and understand life, ourselves, and others, and to do that we must to use all seven emotional lenses proficiently. This means we have to take time to reframe a situation, in order to consider all seven aspects of value instead of just impulsively reacting.

Each emotion is experienced as if through one of the senses. 1) contempt -chills, 2) sadness - sight, 3) surprise - taste, 4) happiness - hearing, 5) anger – touch, muscle tone, 6) fear – stomach churning/twisting, 7) disgust -smell. The general approaches, or fundamental actions which our emotions suggest are: 1) to receive, 2) to refine, 3) to expand, 4) to incorporate, 5) to hold, 6) to take, 7) to give.

We intuitively match emotional lenses through posture, tone and terminology to show openness to connection. This doesn't mean that we should scrutinize our posture or words in response to someone else; the emotional lens is not the only variable in the equation of connection, and it's not one that is easily faked. If we just try to be fully present with someone, we naturally will match their emotion. Since matching emotional lenses is an intuitive action, we likely only notice we are doing it after we have already started. If we don't naturally match emotion there is probably a reason. For example, we are likely to match emotions with a friend who is venting, but less likely with someone who is just complaining.

There is a reason confidence is such an attractive quality and desperateness isn't, because odds are we would rather match someone's confident emotion outlook rather than match their desperate one. It is not a coincidence that when we are single or in the job market, that either no one wants us, or suddenly everyone wants us. Does this mean we should always be confident even if we are unsure? Yes and no... The key is to have positive (productive) emotional states which I call interpersonal tools, and avoid negative (counterproductive or misdirected) emotional states, which I call interpersonal weapons. Of the twenty-one interpersonal tools, confidence is not one, because it is not specific to one emotional lens, it is a component of each tool.

A large step in psychotherapy was the discovery of transference, which is the principle that our neurotic tendencies manifest in pretty much all that we do. By neurotic I mean, certain actions that somehow by-pass our better judgment. Neuroticism doesn't come from a part of us that is trying to sabotage our lives, but rather gaps in our perception that prevent us from being able to make an informed decision. We operate on a combination of assumptions we make, and assumptions others tell us. As we test these assumptions, coincidence and conformation bias are hard to exclude, and so faulty assumptions are not always easily debunked.

Once we feel we have proved an assumption's usefulness, we allow it to operate automatically, like all of the complex movements in walking that we don't think about. Therefore, we have several ideas operating almost completely automatically, which means that the stress they cause is unlikely to be traced back to them, because we don't think about them much when we do them. By reframing a situation, it makes it easier to narrow down and identify the cause of a stress, and challenge the assumptions that lead to it. We have consistent stresses in our live that we have a difficult time pinpointing the source, because we typically frame certain situations in the same way, and neglect to reframe them considering other aspects of value.

When we talk about our problems, our version of the story is obviously flawed, otherwise the solution would be self-evident as we layout the story... our problem is often obvious to those listening to our story, or at least the gapping hole in our narrative is. This discovery of transference allowed therapists to not rely on the stories of their patients, but the way that the patients interact with the therapist. In the lingo of my theory, I would say that our favorite interpersonal tools and favorite interpersonal weapons are the ones we use most often, and that once we discover what our top three favorite weapons are, we will know what has caused almost all the conflict in our life.

The word science comes from the Latin word "scire" which means, "to know." We are born with the tools to understand the world, but not with a readymade understanding of things. This process of understanding things is science, and since life doesn't come with labels or instructions, the only way to understand one thing is to compare and contrast it to another thing. To make the process of comparing and contrasting faster and more efficient, humanity has made an attempt at creating standard for measurements like weight, time, volume and distance.

What to do in a situation is not usually immediately apparent, and so when we do something, what we expected to happen can be quite different from what actually happens. This usually is the case when an aspect of value we didn't consider, was more important than we thought. Though discouraging, when our expectations are undermined by factors we didn't consider, afterwards, we will know to consider them. As we gather this sort of data, we come to understand things to the point that what we expect to happen, happen. We can reduce the gap between what we expect to happen and what actually ends up happening. Essentially that is the definition of science, "conditions of reproducibility."

Frustration comes from undermined "will," and if we make a science of analyzing and testing the interdependence of things, nothing will frustrate us. Stress is strain on our "will," and that cannot be completely avoided, but will abate significantly when we stop pushing against ourselves. Both in testing assumptions, and in recording results, the way that we describe or measure the conditions and the results is very important to improving.

I have an odd example that illustrates quite well what good can come from identifying and standardizing the different aspects of value in life. Technological advancements have been improving at an exponential rate over mainly the last two-hundred years, and it follows a similar course of the process of understanding things better. In the evolution of measurement, doing what seemed most practical, lead to a more profound understanding than anyone could have guess. Weight started as a way to keep prices of simple commodities consistent, and once weight became exact enough, it gave us clues to the fundamental building blocks of life. Likewise, being practical about reframing a situation in seven different aspects of value, leads to a more profound understanding of mind and emotion than we could have guessed.

In 1795, the gram was decreed in France to be "the absolute weight of a volume of pure water equal to the cube of the hundredth part of the metre, at the temperature of melting ice". It is not a coincidence that not to long after precision in measurement was taken seriously, in 1815 Amedeo Avogadro was able to find the connection between the arbitrary measurement of a gram, to how many molecules were in that gram, which has been incredibly useful. In chemistry ratios are very important, for example water, has two hydrogens for every oxygen—because of this, for many reactions, measurements have to be very precise, and weight became the best way to understand and use those ratios.

So why is the history of measurement important? Because just as there are several ways to measure something, weight, height, width, speed, etc, in order to compare and contrast one thing to another, we have seven different aspects of value and criteria of logic to use to compare and contrast one thing to another. In 1999 a spacecraft was created in order to orbit Mars, but because two different companies involved used different measurement systems, this lead to failure of communication with the spacecraft, and it subsequently was lost in space. Similarly, conflict happens between two people when they are both using different emotional lenses, because we will see things pretty differently if we are comparing and contrasting different aspects of value for the same situation.

Measurement of weight has changed over the years since the earliest records of the "deben" which is an Egyptian measurement of weight. Many records from ancient Egypt were about measurements of goods and services than any other thing. Specifically, most records where about measurements of wheat, which started as an arbitrary amount—initially determined by the amount someone could carry or fit into a container someone happened to have, which size then became standard. Today we have weights based on numbers of atoms, or even sub-atomic particles. Similarly, what starts off for us as an arbitrary measurement of stability, safety, functionality, accuracy, continuity, excellence or perspective, as we use those measurements to understand and operate in life, we will find the fundamental units similar to atoms that value and logic are made out of.

We make claims of things regarding aspects of value by giving things descriptor words. Sometimes we say something is best or worst, but don't say in what. This implies that we just assume others are seeing the same aspect of value in it we think is most important. For example, a group deciding where to go to eat, by saying, "I know a good restaurant," one person could strictly mean, "I know an affordable restaurant," meanwhile another person thinks by good they mean "great taste or service." This happens so often, that when some says something is good or best, we have to think about previous occasions they have said something was good and assume they are using the word in the same way. It is often not difficult to guess how someone means "good," or "best" and that shows that we consistently look at things with the same aspect of value, to the point where the influence of our identity (or bias in preferences) often supersedes our language... especially when we don't qualify what we say with adjectives that address objective aspects of value. Trust is fine, and the less important something is, the less needs to be said about it, but because sometimes we don't know what's important to other people, we might as well communicate as best we can... and by best I mean, communicate with the most functionality, accuracy, perspective, continuity, stability, protection and transcendence possible.

When there is a conflict, it is likely that we were not communicating well about one of the interpersonal tools. I have derived these twenty one interpersonal tools from the seven emotional lenses, and I believe that conflict is usually a question about their nature:

Fairness, Forgiveness, Open-mindedness, Kindness, Enthusiasm, Compassion, Appreciation, Teamwork, Prudence, Curiosity, Love, Perseverance, Acceptance, Hope, Leadership, Humility, Creativity, Social intelligence, Honesty, Investigation, Humor.

How do we measure these?

When we tell someone that something wasn't fair, what standard of fairness are we basing that on? When we claim that someone was unkind, what standard of kindness are we measuring with? If the nature of kindness is universal, why is there ever an argument about it? An argument means one person is claiming another person's measurement is wrong—that their measurement better approximates the actual nature of the aspect of value or criteria of logic. This means that theoretically if we all came to a consensus of the nature of aspects of value and criteria of logic, how they compare and contrast, and how to know which is the most important one in each situation, there would be no argument and there would be no conflict. I am not proposing a social movement to achieve that, but merely pointing out what would happen if enough people took this individual journey to explore the objective nature of value and logic.

Just as precision in measurements is one thing that has facilitated many other discoveries in science, so to can understanding the way we measure things improve our ability to understand and navigate through life. When building something, after taking the time to draw up plans, and then taking the time to measure things out, it is pretty nice when the pieces end up actually fitting together. How often are we able to get what was planned in our head to actually happen? Too often our expectations fail us, but if we understand what we are measuring and how to measure, what we plan can materialize.

It's not a matter of just expecting nothing or expecting little, but putting all the tools we are given to form the most accurate and useful expectations. We should make expectations, tons of them, but not hold them so tightly that we break trying to hold them together. Every failed expectation leads to a greater ability to make accurate expectations.

We have a tendency to approach situations the way we feel most comfortable instead of how we think would be best. What we feel comfortable with, is just what we happen to have experience with, which is mostly just what life has thrown at us. We have a choice to let familiarity, or logic and value govern our choices and shape our ideals. The ideals we work towards and taboos we avoid often have more to do with what happens around or to us, than some innate or authentic desire.

We tend to run towards ideals so intensely and avoid taboos so dramatically, that we are so busy running that we miss the subtle innate or authentic thoughts and feelings. That little voice inside of us can't speak as loud as the myriad of opinions pressing on us from all sides. Choosing what opinion is loudest is not the reason to listen, otherwise we will become just an echo of the loudest part of society instead of be what we have potential to be, which is quiet the voice inside us of reason and love.

We get so caught up proving we are ideal and not taboo, that we are distracted from considering what we authentically want to do. Likely experience has suggested to us that what we find value in only has value to us, and even sometimes has negative value to others. This would lead to the logical conclusion that either our ability to sense value is broken, or everyone else's is... which makes it hard not to second guess ourselves, or at least do what we want to do while also showing others what they seem to want to see. The problem with that is that nothing can be completely proved because we can't force someone to consider what we see as facts, especially not an identity, which is not a fact, because everyone sees us differently. We should focus on doing things we see value and logic in whether or not anyone else validates it.

All aspects of value are important in every situation, but one in each situation is pivotal, because the most pivotal aspect of value is the one we use to determine which action to take first in a situation; the order of actions can be important. This is another reason our assumptions of things can be off, is because even having all the right ingredients, using them in the wrong order can still have things fail... leading us to blame the ingredient when it was just the order that was off.

If an action is good, it should be positive or productive in at least one aspect of value, and neutral or positive in the other six. Some things look positive when only seen through one or two aspects of value but are negative in the rest. If someone else is doing something we see no value in, odds are that we are both looking at it with different aspects of value. It's not possible to do something bad for bad's sake, anything we see someone else do at least has one positive aspect of value in that person's mind, whether it is naïve, negligent or not.

Value and logic are two very different things—value often defies logic. Value says that we should jump in the water to save someone drowning because of the value in human life, logic says not to risk losing two lives instead of just one. The order of which aspect of value is most pivotal and least pivotal in a situation changes, but the order of feeling, thinking, and doing doesn't change. Intuition or emotions assess assets or value, and intellect applies logic or reason. We can't apply logic to nothing, the asset is the goal for logical to push towards.

Intuition is non-linear thinking, it suggests where we should go, intellect is linear thinking, it suggests how to get there.

What should happen in the case of a person drowning, is our intuition says it is worth it to save the person, and then our intellect figures out the best way to do it; this might mean throwing some type of flotation device, or jumping in. If we determine that jumping in to save the person has value, that leads to the next application of logic. Do we swim to them from behind like a lifeguard would, so they don't flail and accidently push us under the water, or is it okay to swim directly to them because it's a child that doesn't weigh enough to push us under even if they tried?

Each step isn't something we have to sit down and think about thoroughly, but giving it a second or two could make all the difference. Our intuition works so fast we don't even see what it is doing—it almost immediately gives us an answer of one of seven fundamental actions to take. If we have only one second to act in an emergency situation, it would be best to spend it by letting our intellect determine how to best carry it out, instead of wishing it hadn't happened. Our intuition works much faster than our intellect, but our intellect works much faster than our body's ability to respond, this means we always have at least a split second to think.

If we only listen to our emotions, or only listen to our intellect we are only using half of our potential.

As long as there is more that we don't know than what we do, it is what we don't know that affects us more than what we do know. Actually listening to what our emotions are suggesting helps us tackle what seems like an impossible question: "How do we figure out what we don't know we don't know?"

Once we reframe a situation using each of the emotional lenses, it helps us figure out what we didn't see before through just one lens. It would be hard to explain all of life just by smelling it or just by tasting it. Even just by sight, without any other sense, the world would be pretty confusing.

We are born with all seven emotional lenses, but we have to practice using them. In the beginning phase of learning how to use an emotional lens, we often feel inadequate and would rather avoid that lens and use one we are already better at instead. That means whatever one or two lenses we happened to learn first, are the ones we likely try to use for everything. Just as when learning how to draw as a child, things don't look on paper like they do in our head, the general actions that emotions suggest often look different when we try to carry them out. For example, anger instead of assertiveness which is what it is, looks like aggressiveness. Sadness, instead of accuracy looks more like pessimism.

We can survive without a few emotional lenses, like not being assertive or investigating life, but we can't thrive without them.

Emotions are a communication from our intuition to our intellect, but all too often we use emotions to project them on others—this is opposite of what they are for, and it's no wonder that out of the seven emotions, the English language doesn't even have positive words to describe them. Five out of seven emotions have negative connotations although all seven are neutral.

Our emotions are not trying to create chaos in our life, they are suggesting a general way to approach a situation based on what aspect of value is perceived to be most important. Our intuition perceives value, then suggests a general approach to the intellect which is communicated via an emotion. Then the intellect which perceives logic, identifies the risks, and lastly our will-power formulates and employs a plan. Whether or not our intuition assesses well enough what aspect of value is most pivotal in a situation, ignoring it won't help it get any better. It is best to at least consider how the general approach the emotion was suggesting would play out. What the intuition is basing the general approach on are assumptions, and as our intellect sets logical expectations on those assumptions, they can be challenged and refined. When we try to hold onto our expectations despite reality proving them wrong as the expectations fail, it causes intellectual pain. Trying to guard assumptions from being challenged causes emotional pain.

The intuition sees assets in life like an artist sees potential and wants to add to it. It suggests an approach to a situation by adding. The intuition seeks the type of things we would want written on our gravestone, the things that are taboo to boast about, but that we love being complimented for. The intuition strives to leave a legacy of meaning. It is that feeling that says, "where can I add something of value?"

The intellect on the other hand sees logic like an engineer correlates and then removes risks by eliminating weaknesses. It suggests an approach to a situation by subtracting something. The intellect seeks the things we feel make us capable, and which we use to define ourselves to others as what expertise we have to offer. It is made of the things that merit title, doctor, professor, mechanic, etc, which all remove things, like illness, ignorance, or car problems.

Albert Einstein illustrated the difference between these two mental functions when he said, "The intuitive mind is a sacred gift, and the rational mind is a faithful servant." The intuition adds value, and the intellect performs a service. There are many possible ways of labeling these two functions, the giver and the fixer, the value and logic, or adder and subtractor. Though they are separate functions, we all have both for a reason, and we should help both functions work together.

These two general adding and subtracting functions, apart from their general functions, are specifically seen through each of the emotional lenses—this creates seven different ways to approach a situation by adding, and seven for subtracting. If we don't really think about what to do in a situation, we usually only see two possible approaches. Seeing fourteen possibilities gives us more options, but even better, our will-power has the ability to take the best from the adding and subtracting approaches and form a new plan. The will-power is the executive function, and each time it forms a combination of ideas from the intuition and intellect, both the intuition and intellect are improved by seeing how the two separate things they perceive, value and logic work together.

To find out more that we don't know that we don't know about life and ourselves, we can look into what triggers us about something. If all we know about something is that it triggers us, that means there is something we are not seeing that we could if we look at closer. Contentment has the pre-requisite of gratitude, and composure has the pre-requisite of integrity, but pain has no pre-requisite—this is why it is usually the first part and sometimes the only part of a situation that we perceive. Often it is easier to notice ways that we are conflicting instead of ways we are or could connect.

Though we cannot force it, there are many things we can do to facilitate connection.

There are four pitfalls which separate us from understanding life and connecting with others:

> 1) Entertaining impossibilities
> 2) Distortion from ego-centricity
> 3) Bias towards what we think we can control
> 4) Infatuation with sensations, and personification of ideas.

Bridges can be built over those pitfalls for each situation. Building and crossing these four bridges crosses us over those pitfalls, allowing us to go from the first stage of awareness, victim stage, where connection is not possible, to the fifth stage of awareness where we can fully connect.

We aren't moving backwards or breaking despite how bad off we feel—it is always the case that going back in time to face the problems we had a year ago, we would handle them better. It is easy to be hard on ourselves because we seem to slip and fall, but that is only because the more we become aware of, the more we have to deal with. The saying "ignorance is bliss" isn't the answer. It's too late to go back to being naïve, our only option is to push forward to awareness and understanding.

I hope you will consider what I propose in this book and put it to the test. I believe that your experience, intuition and your own reason will prove my theory valid and useful to have more contentment and composure in your life. I hope the Anatomy of Mind and Emotion helps you as much as it has helped me.

Chapter 1

"I just need a private island and a million dollars, and all my problems would be fixed."

I definitely wouldn't turn down either the island or the million dollars if someone were offering them, but I don't think they would solve the problem. What is the problem?

We want to connect with people, and not just in a networking way—we want to have profound satisfying relationships… and we don't want conflict. I think a big part of the problem is that we want the type of connection we think other people have, so much that we mess up the connection we have… or could have had. Envy isn't the basis of my theory, but the influence of perception, and misdirection of intention that comes from it is important. We don't realize all of the expectations we have silently operating in us that are based on assumptions we pick up from things that look flashy or things that sound catchy, without even thinking about it sometimes.

What we want all too often is undermined by how we expect to get it and what we think will come along with it. It's not that what we want is wrong, we all want to love and be loved, it's just that we have picked up false assumptions about how to love and how to be loved. It's odd how we can genuinely try to love, and still end up heartbroken.

We have likely been a little too hard on ourselves for our love not seeming enough sometimes, but we should cut ourselves some slack. It is unlikely that standing there alone on the playground, in tears after a break-up, or after an argument with someone we love, that we had the solution to human connection which philosophers and poets throughout history have been searching for.

Looking through what has been written about love and connection shows us two things, one, that even the greatest minds in history are about as lost as us when it comes to love, and two, it shows us where we got some of our false assumptions. I think one of the biggest barriers for me as a kid trying to figure out how to make friends and pursue relationships, was the fact that I felt panicked that I had fallen behind, and needed to run to catch up.

It might seem like a lot of quotes, but I hope it will be comforting to know that although people have said many great things about many different topics, when it comes to friendship and connection everyone else including the great minds of history seem to be about as lost as the average one of us. Just like us, writers and public figures were either just as overly optimistic, discouraged or confused. Following the train of thought over the centuries shows how complicated friendship and connection really are. As you read the quotes, see how closely their sentiment matches your experience, and whether they contradict each other.

"A friend is one that knows you as you are, understands where you have been, accepts what you have become, and still, gently allows you to grow." – William Shakespeare

Seneca a first century philosopher had a similar sentiment: "One of the most beautiful qualities of true friendship is to understand and to be understood."

Ralph Waldo Emerson Continues the heart-warming idea: "The glory of friendship is not the outstretched hand, not the kindly smile, nor the joy of companionship; it is the spiritual inspiration that comes to one when you discover that someone else believes in you and is willing to trust you with a friendship."

L.M. Montgomery, who wrote Anne of Green Gables, "True friends are always together in spirit."

Jane Austin, "There is nothing I would not do for those who are really my friends. I have no notion of loving people by halves, it is not my nature."

Maybe Shakespeare, Seneca, Emerson, Austin and Montgomery were exceptionally better at making friends than me. Not to be a cynic, but even as good as some of the friendships I enjoy are, I wouldn't say in every instance I have felt, "accepted and gently allowed to grow," "completely understood," "always together is spirit," or where someone didn't show the limits of how far they would go for me. Maybe your experience has been the same.

It is possible some disappointment is just part of the package deal of friendship. Bob Marley said, "The truth is, everyone is going to hurt you. You just got to find the ones worth suffering for."

If that is true, how then do we know who is worth suffering for? We probably couldn't know who was worth suffering for until we had suffered for them. So maybe we give everyone one chance, and if suffering for them was worth it, we keep them as friends... probably not. Most of my best friends have given me more than one chance, and I have done the same, so I don't think it is that simple.

It would seem logical that whomever accepts and understands us the best, would be the person to be friends with, right? Maybe... but wouldn't that be quite the double-standard. It doesn't seem very accepting if we only accepted someone if they accepted us first.

Apart from being a fairly selfish motive to only accept people into our life that accept us first, and only take the time to get to know people that have already taken the time to get to know us, it also provokes the questions, "How well do we even know ourselves?"

The questions, "How many people truly know us? How many people do we truly know?" don't make very much sense if we don't know ourselves very well.

Maybe how well we know ourselves is a limit to how well we can know someone else. Or maybe the opposite, how well we know someone else is the limit to how well we can know ourselves. Noticing what someone else does well or ought to change is a lot easier than realizing what we do well or can change... but then again, experiencing the benefit or consequence of our own action poignantly brings something to our attention that would have appeared meaningless watching someone else do it. In short, actions have consequences, some that are easier to see in ourselves, and others that are easier to see in others, and whichever one we notice first, we should look to see if it is consistent with the other's experience.

Chapter 2

There has been a recent push to make mental health something people can talk about instead of suffering in silence. Mental health implies that there is a normal or healthy that we are trying to get back to. I think it is not a matter of mental health but mental maturity. In the preface and introduction I outlined the twenty-one interpersonal tools, and considering that in the context of mental maturity, we all learn different tools at different times. It is impossible to be perfectly proficient with an interpersonal tool, and I have not met anyone that was considerably proficient with all the tools, therefore, there is no way to determine who is overall more psychologically mature.

I won't name names, but one company in particular, I find it interesting that every other product I really enjoy, but the ones in between, I'm not sure why they did so many random new things that aren't as good as the way things were in older versions. Does this mean that the company alternates between being sick and being healthy for the last few decades? No, it's just that growth comes from innovation, but not all innovation leads to growth.

Mental maturity is similar, we are learning and growing, and since both are so difficult to measure, that when we try, sometimes we come to the conclusion that we are moving backwards, that we are mentally ill…. When we are not—it's likely just new territory. This isn't to say that mental illness doesn't exist, but that much of what the average person may think is mental illness is just an innovative step that is awkward, not a disease. I remember the first time I felt growing pains in my legs, I was scared there was something wrong with me— really I was just growing. I have female friends that had no idea what a menstrual cycle was until they were bleeding and terrified.

I think that too often we are frozen in fear when faced with mental growing pains to see and enjoy the fact that we are growing. I think we become blinded by shame, guilt and fear, and that only makes the growing process slower. This book is Anatomy of Mind and Emotion, not anatomy of shame, guilt and fear, but how are we supposed to map out our mind and emotion is we are too scared and embarrassed to look at ourselves deeply?

We're not sick, and we've not broken, we are developing proficiency with different interpersonal tools, and it's not a straightforward process, so we should cut ourselves some slack. We all have interpersonal tools we are good with and ones we are not, and I believe that a big reason why we are not good at some interpersonal tools is because of a strong taboo on their associated weapon, it makes it difficult to get close enough to figure them out. We become so sensitive and disgusted with the idea of lying for example, that we feel so obligated to be forthcoming and transparent, but know that it comes at a cost. The definition of deceit in that case has encroached on the definition of honesty, making our focus primarily on avoiding dishonest instead of figuring out how to proficiently use honesty. (Refer to the preface for more on that tool.)

For this reason, understanding shame, guilt and fear must be discussed first, so that the strong taboos we have don't prevent us from understanding what valuable things they are associated with. Shame, guilt, and fear have the ability to keep us distracted almost incessantly if we let them, and being distracted make it hard to learn and grown.

We shouldn't feel scared to look inside ourselves, we aren't going to find the metaphorical "skeletons in our closet" that people talk about, what we will find, are defense mechanisms working automatically trying to keep us "safe." Ironically, our defense mechanisms are what cause most of our conflicts, but because they are mindless processes, they don't know they are really fighting against themselves. For this reason, we just need to debunk the vague idea of "safe" that involves safe from possible shame, guilt and fear, because we shouldn't be ashamed, guilty or fear growing pains.

Our mental immaturity is room we have to grow, it's a seed that hasn't grown, not a the skeleton remains of something that was alive before. If we look at our immaturity as a skeleton in our closet, that will mean that we will have to find some reason to love ourselves in spite of the reasons not to.

We can only appreciate others to the extent in which we appreciate ourself. If we deficiently appreciate ourselves, it would be hard to believe that another person could truly appreciate us, and vice versa. The more we know, the more there is to appreciate.

When I say "know," I mean concerning things of objective nature. Objective means a conclusion that can be confirmed by someone else because it is real. For example, in science, where, when the conditions of an experiment are replicated, the results are replicated as well.

There is one thing we learn but can't understand, because it is not objective, and that is shame, guilt and fear. Neither of those three can constantly be reproduced when replicating what produced them in someone else. This isn't to say that they aren't "real" because when we talk about something like shame, we are lumping in the actual chemical changes that accompany certain ways of thinking with influence of how we imagine other people see us, or the subjective way we see ourselves. Duty and empathy are a real or objective consequence of recognizing how an action we have done negatively affects someone else, but becomes subjective or not real when we add in what we imagine that action does to our image.

We are not an image or an identity, we are a self in a world of actual things of objective nature having a subjective experience. It was thousands of years, till somewhat recently that anyone knew the purpose or function of the appendix which is attached to our intestines. We now know much more about it now, about the immunological cells that reside there, but we don't know everything. The more we learn about the actual nature of something, the more objective it becomes, and the better we can interact with it. This is important, because that means that there is no definitive endpoint for learning. This means that without a perfectly objective understanding of something, we couldn't interact with it perfectly, hence why every action is a learning opportunity.

All too often we look at what we do as either successful or not—this polarization leads to us feeling like a failure or a success. In reality, with each thing we do, there is at least some part worth repeating, and some part not worth repeating.

The root of shame is the subjective assumption that we are objectively wrong or bad. Shame is assuming our self-worth is too low to be worth connecting to. We should want to rectify what we do that negatively affects other people, but that should be an enabling motivation of duty and empathy, not the disabling feeling of shame. There is a lingering uncertainty of whether our efforts to rectify our mistakes with others will be enough, or be accepted, but all we can do is our best, there is no point on ruminating on it.

We are often so scared to make mistakes, but realizing we have made a mistake increases our ability to connect. Trying to rectify mistakes brings us closer because when we try to fix something, we are centering our efforts on another person, and facilitating the conversation that rarely happens. This often produces a conversation where we ask what we can do to help, and someone shares what they really think and feel. It is our desire to connection that brings an authentic conversation, not the panging emotional pain of shame. We should make "I'm sorry," to mean, "I want to understand and rectify," instead of, "I'm embarrassed I mess up."

When we try to rectify a mistake, that duty we feel inside pushes us to step outside of ourselves and to focus on what someone else thinks and feels. Shame is where we hide inside of ourselves to not face what we have done on the outside. This does not mean we let someone rule over us under the pretense that we wronged them, it means we try to do what we can in order to better see from their point of view.

The feeling of shame distracts us from analyzing and remembering what is worth repeating or emulating and what is not. If repeating or emulating something will likely bring the feeling of shame, it might not seem worth it even if it actually is. This is why we sometimes don't want to reach out to other people or take responsibility when we know we should.

It is hard to ignore the presence of shame and try to be objective about understanding the value and risks of things. How often do we feel anxious about telling the truth because we know there will be repercussions?

How many times have we tried to weigh out in our minds the consequences of lying because we don't think someone can handle the truth? How often do we not own up to mistakes we have made because we would rather rectify them in secret rather than having our mistake be rationale for others shaming us? "I didn't break it, but I will help you fix it," gets us more praise and less drama than, "I broke it, but I will help fix it," so what incentive is there to be honest?

It is sad that much of what we fear happening and are embarrassed of are accidents. We are even sometimes embarrassed for completely normal and almost unavoidable things like coughing or sneezing.

"I didn't break it, but I will help fix it," means that we can spend less time and energy dealing with the drama and more time and energy helping fix the thing... unless later the truth is found out. There is a reason why we avoid people, or are careful what we do with certain people—it's because dealing with the damage we cause ourselves with our own mistakes is hard enough without possibly adding more.

When we forgive someone, we get to exercise our ability to show compassion which feels good, therefore we have no reason to suspect that other people don't also feel good when they forgive others. I have found that people often are more willing to forgive others than they are to forgive themselves. When we try to rectify our mistakes that affect others, we can show compassion by really trying to understand the other person. "I'm sorry, please forgive me," all too often sounds like, "I'm embarrassed I got caught." Empathy would sound something like, "I have come to realize that you must have felt _____ when I did/didn't _____, and I feel if I were you, that me doing _____ would help to rectify it. I now see the value in _____ which I didn't see before. I want you to feel free to tell me how you feel about what happened, and I want you to know I am invested in making it right."

We aren't born with perfect awareness, learning to notice what is around us is a process. What complicates that process is that we have two separate parts of are mind working almost completely independently. Part of our thinking is intuitive or unconscious, which means we don't see happening, and part of our thinking is intellectual which we do see happening. "Why did you do that?" can honestly be met with, "I don't know?" because our intuition doesn't have words to describe it or logic behind what it wants to do. The intuition communicates, but non-verbally. Intuition manifests in our posture, our breathing, our heartrate, and anything we don't consciously control. This is why when people are really good friends, seeing an emotion manifesting from the outside is almost as easy to understand and being the one feeling the emotion. Especially in a child, where they are feeling an emotion for the first time, an observer, like a parent, can pick up on what the child is feeling and articulate it before the child has figure out what they are feeling, and long before they could find a way to articulate it.

Similarly to how coughing or sneezing can seem more like a source of embarrassment, so also we often neglect to treat emotions as useful part of us. It is a bigger task that it seems to simultaneously become aware of what can be expressed in words, and what can't. If you've ever given someone a hug and had them collapse in your arms with a sigh, you know how much can be said without any words. Because of the difficultly trying to become aware of two almost completely separate worlds, one of words and one of emotion, in the journey of psychological maturity, we often focus more on one than the other.

We stumble our way through both worlds the one described with words that is concerned with results and logic, and the other without words to describe it, that is concerned with intent and meaning. We learn the physical nature of things, and the world of meaning or intent imposed on physical things. We learn that a dollar bill holds some extra significance that a different similar shaped piece of paper has. We learn that spilling a cup of juice on the dirt has the physical consequence of not getting to drink it, and then learn that spilling a cup of juice on the carpet has an extra consequence above forgoing being able to drink it.

We learn that apart from science there is ethics, and that some scientific studies like those Hitler performed in WWII logical or not, we're unethical. Sometimes with equal disgust we stumble into things that are ethical but not logical. It is an odd experience to stumble into something that is only part of one world and not the other—that something has logic but no meaning or vice versa. It is unsettling to feel the need to not only balance but optimize both worlds, that of meaning and that of logic. The reason the riddle of life is so difficult to solve, is because it is nether world, the one of logic nor the one of meaning, but that space where they overlap. It seems the most common way we become aware of those worlds, aware of ourselves as part of those worlds, and aware of the people and things that surround us, is by stumbling or crashing into them.

It is a lot easier to learn when we stumble into physical things, but when there is accompanying pain, it can be very distracting. There have been a number of people who have a bee or wasp fly in their car window when driving, and then let the pain, or even just the fear of the sting makes them lose focus on the road and crash. Whether there is an actual sting in love and connection or not, we shouldn't crash our car over it.

C.S. Lewis, in The Four Loves says, "To love at all is to be vulnerable. Love anything and your heart will be wrung and possibly broken. If you want to make sure of keeping it intact you must give it to no one, not even an animal. Wrap it carefully round with hobbies and little luxuries; avoid all entanglements. Lock it up safe in the casket or coffin of your selfishness. But in that casket, safe, dark, motionless, airless, it will change. It will not be broken; it will become unbreakable, impenetrable, irredeemable. To love is to be vulnerable."

We can't control how other people will react, but we can control what we do. There is a blurry line between being recklessly vulnerable and open to connection, but connection is not possible without vulnerability. Since the enlightenment era the world of logic has seemed like less of a gamble than the world of meaning, because logic increasingly became predictable, but that came at the expense of people doing what seemed crazy.

For example, what did Isaac Newton think he was going to logically find by meticulously charting the stars for several years? But he found quite a bit. Concerning love and connection, for some of us we may think or feel that the craziest or most risky part is the logic while for others the meaning; whichever it is for us, it's okay to feel a little bit crazy.

The author of Alice and Wonderland, Lewis Carroll said, "You're mad, bonkers, completely off your head. But I'll tell you a secret. All the best people are."

Aristotle agreed, "No great mind has ever existed without a touch of madness."

There are things in life that happen, that if we didn't know they were common would make us think we were crazy. Where do incredibly random but still very vivid dreams come from? Or how does sleep walking happen? Where do cravings come from? And why does music have an effect on us?

Possibly the most puzzling question is, why do we not like some of our own thoughts or feelings? Why do we think or feel things if we don't like them? Are they us? Or are we just along for the ride they are carrying us on? Are we the one's commentating on random thoughts that generate, or are we the thoughts and something else is commentating on them? I will not attempt to explain the phenomenon of dreams anymore than to say that they possibly give us symbolic directions, and also somewhat indicate the stage of awareness we are in for a given principle or situation. The stages of awareness in a dream could be on a spectrum from being chased, fighting, doing, and then to flying. I will explain the stages of awareness later, but not how they correlate to dreams, because dreams are not the focus of this book, and it is the most recent and therefore least substantiated part of my theory. I bring up the topic of dreams merely to point out a line between conscious and unconscious processes in our minds. I draw this line so I will be able to then draw a line in the unconscious, separating what is real, or us, in other words, the permanent components, and what parts of our unconscious are merely transitory.

It is unlikely that what we call insanity is a conscious process. In my experience working in inpatient and outpatient psychiatry, I never met an insane person who knew they were being insane. It would follow that what we call insanity is relegated to the unconscious part of the mind. Also, because even the clinically insane seem to wax and wane in lucidity, it is unlikely that insanity is in the formal or permanent part of the unconscious which is the intuition. Insanity is in the temporary unconscious processes like triggers and reflexes, which can undermine our better thinking.

I have found that either real or imagined, each bout of insanity large or small seems to have someone or something it is fighting against. This emergency status situation I think gives the reflexive defense mechanisms conscious permission. "I was trying to hold it together, but then I just lost my cool and blew up on them," is how sometimes an event is described; giving conscious support for the need to lose control, and minimizing whatever actions happened as a defense mechanism to "blew up on them."

It is a scary thought that there could be process outside of our direct conscious control that negatively affect our lives. This could lead us to fear our unconscious and try to confine it. When what we should confine, are our triggers and reflexes, we sometimes try to confine our whole unconscious including our emotions... leading to both the emotions and defense mechanisms bursting out at once. The question is, is it possible to leave our unconscious mind unchecked and eliminate the triggers? Is there some dividing line between the unconscious negative motives and unconscious positive motives?

It sure feels unnatural to not be able to completely control our mind or emotions, but is it even possible to control them completely? Or is it even necessary?

Edgar Allan Poe suggested in the book, The Tell-tale Heart, "It is impossible to say how first the idea entered my brain; but once conceived, it haunted me day and night." And on another occasion said, "I was never really insane except upon occasions when my heart was touched."

That is a kind of terrifying prospect, that an idea can haunt us. If true, this would give us reason to fear our unconscious mind. If the unconscious part of our mind is a monster, or can be corrupted into being one, how could we stop it?

Friedrich Nietzsche suggested the ideas infecting the mind started in the heart. "One ought to hold on to one's heart; for if one lets it go, one soon loses control of the head too."

It is a terrifying thing to think there is something wrong with our mind or with our heart. The most debilitating thing is thinking that our heart or mind is broken or infected, because what would we use to fix it? If there is something wrong with our mind, how would our mind be able to find or fix it? And to have people like Edgar Allan Poe and Friedrich Nietzsche telling us that the ideas we have are just the ones strong enough to haunt us, or that if we let our heart do what it wants to do for even a moment that we could go insane.

Are we our thoughts and emotions?

Albert Camus offered his insight, "Man is the only creature who refuses to be what he is." If true, this would mean that all our ideas and feelings are our own, that we are both the random ideas and feelings, and the commentator that despises them.

So, who do we trust, Poe? Nietzsche? Camus?

What we think we are, makes a pretty big difference in how we should go about doing things. An opposing idea to Poe, Nietzsche and Camus is that we have control over how we process the random thoughts and feelings, that we can decide how we put them into action, and who we are is that ever-changing part inside us that chooses actions and can learn from them.

What I like to do is consider all the options. Put them all up on the table, and then compare and contrast them with each other, with my own experience, and with other things. Using biology as a model sheds some light on what the two possible options of the nature of the unconscious mind are: Either our mind and emotions are susceptible to a type of cancer or just as we transitioned through many different stages that don't resemble the end goal until we are almost there—like a fetus which passes through many stages that don't look at all human. Likewise, our mind and emotions are growing and won't resemble what they are supposed to until they almost are what they should or could be.

The other idea is that the touch of insanity in us is like a cancer, an infection, or an awkward stage of development. Insanity could therefore either be like a cancer, where something in our unconscious has gone rogue because it mutated, like an infection because it is something foreign trying to take us over, or insanity might just be a result of an awkward stage in development where certain functions aren't functional yet.

Just as we are born without every biological function working, it is possible that that our mind and emotions are also not done developing. For example, the sex characteristics, which begin to mature after roughly eight years—drastically changing body development and presence of hormones. Maybe emotional or intellectual maturity is something that take at least that long, or maybe much longer. My conclusion is that it is the later. Just as a uterus in preparation to create offspring each month creates a new lining and sheds it if not needed, similarly even once emotional or intellectual maturity is reached, there still are inconvenient and unpleasant things that happen, some kind of emotional or mental period.

How do we separate growing pains from inherent inconveniences and unpleasantness that randomly happen in life? Or are they both just mixed together?

Claude Monet said, "Color is my daylong obsession, joy, and torment." What Monet chose to do with the chaotic amalgamation of obsession, joy and torment, which color was to him, he chose to paint it in the best way possible.

Wolfgang Amadeus Mozart suggests that the obsession, joy and torment of something that captures us might be born of our own love. "Neither a lofty degree of intelligence nor imagination nor both together go to the making of genius. Love, love, love, that is the soul of genius."

Is it that we plant seeds of thought, and that as those seeds grow, they change, and drop other seeds? If so, how are we to know from the looking at a mere seed what will grow? That brings us back to the possibly of our hearts and minds being infected, because we can't possibly conceive what will become of each little thing we do. For example, a friend nine years ago asked me where my outlook on life met with psychology...

A study of history and philosophy, classes on neuroscience, four years of bio-chemistry, then four more of medical school, and a pile of psychology literature later, and here I am writing a book... I don't know if my friend is to blame for infecting me, or that she merely awoke what would have bloomed at some point anyway, but it is now my obsession, joy and torment, and I am totally okay with that. It's not like she was the only one to ask me a question that made me think, and if this idea has outcompeted the others, maybe it just has more value to me than the rest. Not to mention, if I wanted to steer my mind another way, I could just find a more intriguing question to ask myself.

Now looking back, it wasn't really just one infecting idea, it was many.

For me, it probably started while standing on a raft in the middle of a pond at eight years old at a camp out, and having several kids on the shore start throwing rocks at me for no reason. I remember wondering why someone would do something cruel like that, and how they even could seem to enjoy it. Although maybe, even without either of those events of people throwing rocks or questions at me, I would have inevitably got to the same place.

All the quotes I have included so far are mostly just to bring up the fact, that life is not a riddle that has been solved yet, and whether we are standing there on a raft in the middle of a pond with rocks splashing all around us, or with a faded and torn pair of movie tickets someone special gave us that we still haven't used because life took us in different directions, we shouldn't beat ourselves up for not having the answer. The great thing about being infected with questions that haunt us, is we are motivated to find answers that enrich and sustain us.

We are not broken, life is not impossible, it just takes a serious study of the questions as they come. The questions we are struggling with are questions that have been brought up over and over again throughout history, and not definitively answered, but we have the advantage of all the pieces of answers that have already been found till now.

Chapter 3

Aristotle said, "Wishing to be friends is quick work, but friendship is a slow ripening fruit." So maybe eight, or even eighteen is way too young to expect to really have a profound and unfailing friendship... especially a friendship like the one he talked about when he said, "What is a friend? A single soul dwelling in two bodies."

Merging two businesses often requires a team of people and is not quick work, even if the assets and liabilities are already delineated by accountants and lawyers. In the venture of "merging souls" as Aristotle put it, where the assets are not really known until long after the merge is over, is much more of a feat. How is this feat managed?

Friedrich Nietzsche suggests, "Love is blind; friendship closes its eyes." So maybe the answer is a matter of just stop looking into things so much. Nietzsche must have been on the same page as Helen Keller who said, "I would rather walk with a friend in the dark, than alone in the light."

One would think, that something so essential to life as friendship would have more insight on it than is currently written, or that it would even at least point in the same direction. Mahatma Gandhi proposed that friendship was so essential that the world depended on it. "With every true friendship, we build more firmly the foundations on which the peace of the whole world rests."

Or, maybe less is written on friendship because it is not actually needed to survive, and we are so busy trying to survive, we don't often get the luxury of true friendship. "Friendship is unnecessary, like philosophy, like art.... It has no survival value; rather it is one of those things which give value to survival."
– C.S. Lewis

So maybe the question of the ages is, "How do we prevent all that is necessary to survive get in the way of what it means to thrive?"

Thomas Fuller said, "If you have one true friend, you have more than your share."

If what Fuller said is at all accurate of the norm, I would say in that case that I am very lucky. It still begs the question, even if we have experienced a friendship that has already grown to be a fairytale refuge from the storm and a treasure greater than gold, why is it probably still not stress-free?

It is possible that the biggest obstacle in the process of psychological maturation, is limited possible measurements— A simple "yes" or "no" or, "good" or "bad" are not measurements.

Things are not polarized or opposites, if we have only two categories for things, we will only have two ways to approach them, completely support and completely reject. This makes what seems like a grey area between the two become erratic as we find it difficult to settle on whether it is good or bad. Seeing things polarize is more reactive and less useful than seeing things for what each part is compared and contrasted individually to everything else we know.

What do the labels we put on things show about how we see them? "Thing I like," "Thing I don't like," is liable to change radically from the one label to the other, leaving us lost when it changes. If we look at something through only one emotional lens or aspects of value, it is likely that we will find out it is not what we thought. If we look at something through all seven emotional lenses it is unlikely we will find we were wrong about all of them at the same time, and so even when one changes, we are still grounded in the other six. We are more likely to make steady progress when we have some consistency in our perception of the life.

Labeling things in reference to stress or shame is not a very effective or stable system for labeling the world. Obvious freedom from stress or shame would be ideal, but in our rush to try to put a label on everything, we should consider the purpose of labeling. If there are only two categories, "causes stress," and "doesn't cause stress," it's only a matter of time before we will have switched the label back and forth so many times we give up on the whole system. The question is not whether someone causes stress, but whether the stress is worth it.

We can calculate or measure the value and the risks of things to the best of our ability, and then if it seems worth it, do it. After we carry out and action, we can see how closely our measurement system predicted the actual value and risks, and then adjust them accordingly. We likely are more capable of measuring or assessing certain aspects of value rather than others, and how we became proficient with the ones we use well, is comparing predicted and actual value and risks after an action is made. There are seven aspects of value, and we are likely only proficient with two or three, therefore the reactivity, or confusion and stress come from the other four or five we are not proficient with measuring.

As we look at life, things first appear as either an asset or a risk, and as our understanding matures, we see in each case how there is an asset, and it has its attached risks. We also see how each asset apart from gaining associated risks, gains more or deeper assets as we understand more about it. For each person there are too many assets and too many risks to count.

If we want to grow, and growing pains are inevitable, a good friend would not be someone who shields us from growth in order to help us avoid pain, but supports us when it comes. Who also isn't scared to tell us for the truth when we ask for it, or motivate us to ask when we don't want to. A good friend is someone who loves us as a person more than the benefits of our friendship as a business deal. There are times when what feels right, might risk the friendship, but trusting that someone is strong enough to handle the truth is a great compliment, and caring enough to be honest with as much compassion possible is a great gesture.

It seems odd to say, "I love you more than our friendship, and to love you I am willing to risk losing our friendship." But imagine the opposite, "I love our friendship more than I love you, and I am willing to risk losing you in order to keep our friendship." It's not very clear-cut though, though we should be willing to give up the business deal benefits of a friendship for the welfare of our friend, it also makes it is more difficult to invest towards the welfare of someone without having a friendship with them. This is an instance of balancing and optimizing the two world, the logic of the friendship, and the meaning of the individual. Both logic and meaning push and pull on each other, and being aware of that effect helps us avoid it undermining the purpose of friendship.

Two heads are better than one, for both understanding and denial, depending on which we choose.

Henry David Thoreau said, "True friendship can afford true knowledge. It does not depend on darkness and ignorance."

There must be a time and a place for eyes wide open and eyes shut in friendship, it can't just be one or the other. I would propose that it depends on whether seeing was the important part for a given situation. Sometimes we should close our eyes and listen to the music, enjoy a scent, or savor a taste, other times we need to really take a good look at the things around us.

Chapter 4

If your experience is anything like mine, part of the stress of making and keeping friends, is that we feel like we should already know how to do it, which adds an additional disappointment to a conflict of any magnitude in a friendship. The fact that it doesn't come naturally when it seems like it should, adds the extra stress of wondering if it is because there is something wrong with us. We replay conflicts in our mind, and play out in advance interactions that might happen.

How much of our time is spent saying something in our heads and trying to imagine how someone will respond, versus just saying it and finding out?

When we imagine a conversation in our minds, we are likely to be critical of it, otherwise we wouldn't feel the need to rehearse it. The idea that we can rehearse or practice an interaction before it happens leads to the idea that we can perfect something before we say it, which both is impossible and has the likely natural consequence of consciously or sub-consciously questioning why others haven't perfected what they say.

The purpose of speaking is to convey something in our mind to someone else. It is an invite for others to be part of our inner-life, and for them to invite us in return. The objective of conversation is to listen for understanding. If the understanding doesn't come, then questions can be asked; there really isn't any point in criticizing what someone says. All criticism does is deter someone from inviting us into the inner-life of their mind. If we listen in order to learn, appreciate and understand, then we will know how to best share our insight with someone else. People can have differing opinions and still listen for understanding.

We shouldn't try to imagine what someone else would think of our inner-life, or try to find a way to dress up our words so our inner-life sounds more interesting, but simply open up to others and see what they think and feel, and appreciate opportunities when others do the same. If our inner-life consists of trying to do the best our judgement is capable of, likely others will see some value in what we have done, and be interested to see what inside of us produced it. Opening ourselves up to others often leads to others opening up to us, and through this, we both see things in others that we would want to change in ourselves. Sometimes it is easier to see something of value or something that is a risk in others that we have been oblivious in ourselves, and it can lead to change.

We often narrate how we feel about what we experience almost as if we were an observer of our own thoughts and emotions—this is neither good nor bad, but how we do narrate can make quite a difference. For example, it would be odd to narrate a story without mentioning the hero, or not mentioning the villain. There is a reason we like to read a story with certain story arch of the hero's journey, and we should narrate our life the same.

Logic has words to describe it, value or meaning can only be described as a journey. This means there should be two distinctly different commentators, one processing thoughts and feelings as logic, and the other processing them as a story or journey.

Some things are better to narrate more light-heartily because there is not much we can change about them anyway, and other things are better to narrate more seriously. What we say about our experience become a precedence for how we will feel in future experiences. For better or worse, a precedence can send us into action a lot faster and with increased chances that we will do something we wouldn't have done had we thought about it more. This affects other people and it also affects ourselves, because we set precedence how we treat others or ourselves in certain situations.

Shaming is a common way we approach subversion of expectations or disappointment, in both how we commentate on other people's actions and our own, and both effect each other negatively. The negative self-talk instills mistrust in ourselves and in others because if our positive intentions are undermined by negative ones, then positive in other people we will assume also is or will be undermined by some negative we don't see. The negative judgments on others creates a harsher and more impossible standard for ourselves. All negative talk is unproductive.

Our internal narration sets the tone for what we look for, which determines what we will see and experience. If we look for something disappointing we will probably find it. If we look for something positive, or better something that we can make more positive, we will likely find it. If we can't see the positive in a situation, or what someone says, we should remember, it's okay to not know something yet. Not knowing doesn't mean we should feel shame, it means we stumbled into something we didn't know we didn't know... but now that we know what it is that we didn't know, we can start to figure it out.

Figuring out life and connection are quite extensive tasks, which will likely be a lifelong journey to complete. If the greatest minds recorded in history haven't settled the nature of connection or life, we should beat ourselves up for not having solved it either.

Apart from the task being difficult, we have likely been told wrong ideas about life and connection, namely the lie that we have to make ourselves worth connecting to. From that lie comes the fear that anything we might do or might have done, can make us unworthy of connection.

We are born with awareness, imagination and will-power, and combined with any other awareness, imagination and will-power both will be increased; that is the value of connecting. What we are born with is all we have and all need to give. You were born worthy of connection, don't ever second guess it!

In my own life, I thought I was fighting shame by making myself more interesting, when really fighting the idea of shame made it stronger and feel more real. Not to mention fighting shame wasted time and energy I could have used in finding things that were interesting for their own sake, and not just as a means to get rid of shame. Feeling ashamed of myself made me less willing to open up, which ironically made it harder to connect.

Being interesting in someone else despite their imperfections helps others and ourselves feel confident in opening up, instead of feeling that we have to hide if we aren't perfect. If we took the time we spend trying to hide and spent it looking for good and trying to make it better, we would make things better for ourselves and everyone around us.

Dale Carnegie in his book, How to Win Friends and Influence People, said, "You can make more friends in two months by becoming interested in other people than you can in two years by trying to get other people interested in you."

That book would have helped quite a bit when I was young...

Gary Chapman author of the Five Love Languages echoes Carnegie's idea, "Love is something you do for someone else, not something you do for yourself."

Wait... does that mean love and connection are paradox? Shouldn't connection be both people being interested in each other? And how do we find the motivation to be interested in someone else without factoring in that love we give to others will be returned to us?

Does one person just have to prime the pump to get it started, and be the first one to take interest?
What if they never take interest back?

I think one of the reasons it took me so long to figure out the answer to my question, was because the answer doesn't seem to make sense. If we care about someone so that they will care about us, it's no more than an unspoken business agreement. And if we just love because love feels good, really we just love, love, and people are just the medium.

What I realized, was that the important question was not how to connect with others, but whether I was willing or not to open myself up for it, to reach out, even if no one ever reached back. Because connection is a choice, this is how we can have our eyes open and shut at the same time. We look to see what good we can add to, and close our eyes to the condition that anything is paid back in return. We have two sets of eyes, one that sees value and the other that sees logic, and it's a matter of closing on set of eyes while seeing with the other, then switching. Just as our two legs are different and walking happens smoothest when a step with the right leg follows a step with the left, likewise connection comes best we take a step with our heart, and then a step with our mind. We likely don't remember not knowing how to walk, but I imagine the process is similarly awkward but possible.

There are many indirect benefits of choosing to be open for connection, which only come after we chose to open ourselves for connection. For example, it is very liberating to see everyone, and know that no one owes you anything, and you don't owe anyone else anything, because that's not how life works. When we look at what possibly could be owed, we will stop seeing people, and only see good employees or bad ones. It is very draining to be promoting, demoting or firing people from our lives when they don't hold up the unspoken deal of expectations.

When we see an asset in life, we have two choices, try to take it, or try to add to it. When this is our focus, we get to pick which assets we are most excited to add to, and not have to worry about auditing debts. People are more inclined to be okay with us finding something they are already doing that we want to support, then us trying to make them do something different.

As a kid I caught a kangaroo rat in the dessert and took him home. I didn't realize how much the arid environment he was used to mattered... over time his fur stopped being as dry as it was when I found him, and I think he was getting sick. What I have found in life, is that some things just can't be taken from where they are and remain the same.

A friend enables us to be best person we can be, by supporting us in the good we are trying to do and inspiring us to notice more. Friends don't make changes in each other, they accelerate changes, there's a difference.

Something interesting I realized, is that each time the question of connection occurred to me, it was because I wanted others to do something. After changing my approach and really trying to figure out what others were doing first, before imposing what I wanted them to do, I found there actually was quite a bit about what they were already doing that I wanted to help with. Before I knew it, I was connecting.

It can seem sometimes like everyone wants something from us, and it's refreshing when someone doesn't want anything from us, when someone just appreciates that we are us. If is beautiful when there is something we are doing that someone else sees as valuable enough of an asset that they want to participate in making it better. If the most detrimental lie circulating is that we must be worthy of connection otherwise there is something wrong with us, then the most helpful thing we can do is validate someone's ability to see and do things of value, and proving the value we see by investing in it.

We don't have the time nor the energy to invest in everything someone does, and we shouldn't either. We should simply look for the best someone is doing, and then validate and support it, not different than we do with ourselves. We shouldn't validate all of the raw thoughts and feeling that pass through us, but focus on the best ones, and then go from there.

Not wanting anything from someone means that we want them to stay the same, it is that we know they already have or will have things they want to change for themselves; we can support where we can, and help when asked. "I don't want anything from you, except that I hope you know I am here if you ever need anything," should be a lot more common of a phrase than it is.

This might seem contradictive, to say that we don't want someone to do something, but then tell others to feel free to ask things of us. Wanting someone to do something and asking someone to do something are two very different things. One carries an expectation and the other opens up possibilities.

Asking someone to do something after they have established they want you to ask, is not totally necessary, but in many cases, is a lot more effective.

I think another reason not wanting someone to be something or do something is unproductive, is that the pressure we add to what they should do makes it difficult to see things unbiasedly. What to do is already a hard enough decision, therefore, adding on who will be disappointed and who will be happy depending on what we do makes it even harder.

If we think that something has value on its own, then the other person should be able to see that same value—we don't need to force them to do it. If we have some insight about someone's choice, we should ask them first what they hope from their choice. Then if the insight we have could help them get what they already want, they we can ask if they would like our insight.

I was talking with someone, and they said they hated using their insulin for their type 2 diabetes. This was not in a clinic setting, and so I asked what they didn't like about it and how much they didn't like it. I then asked if they had tried any other options. They said no. I asked if they would like my insight. They said they did, and I explained about the correlation between better diet and insulin in our body. I answered questions, and I didn't try to get any sort of commitment out of them, because I didn't want them to feel obligated to me to do it. I knew that it has value in itself.

I found that it was something they already wanted, and appreciated the insight I gave, because quickly they lost weight, and then excitedly told me how their doctor had told them they no longer need insulin. This was the first time I have seen someone do that, and I think it was because I was listening, and noticed the opportunity to support them in what they already wanted to do.

It is very easy to make it seem like us and the thing we want someone to be or do are a package deal, and that they have to accept or reject them us and the thing we want them to do. This distorts us and the thing we want that person to do, because they won't be able to see either for what it is on its own. I think that is why we are selective about who we connect with, because we are scared of everything else that is attached to each person, their taboos and ideals they will impose on us.

In sense, I think often we are too smart to simply enjoy life. One of the strongest connections is a parent and their newborn child. There's no excuse that we are not as cute as we were when we were born, with our little fingers and toes, and that funny look of surprise on our infant face of "what the heck just happened?" when we were born. We are born helpless, needy, and crying, and with nothing to offer by our presence, but for some reason it is more than enough—the connection is palpable.

It is sad and ironic that likely we felt appreciated and loved when we were helpless and crying, and now we feel we have to be capable and confident to be worth connecting to. The first time I watched a baby be born I cried. The first time I delivered a baby, right as the baby slid into my hands, I felt what seemed to be an electric shock—I was completely overpowered with awe. I felt the connection to that adorable little infant that I didn't even know and knew I would likely never see again.

We are all born with what we need to connect, which is just us. I saw many assets in that infant, all the possible things that child would grow up to do. I saw the one thing that baby was focused on doing, that was just being alive, and breathing, and I saw how I could support them, and I did—that is when I felt the connection. Why should it be any harder to see what someone else is trying to do? Aren't we all just trying to be alive and to breath? Are we all just trying to live and love and be love? And won't holding someone almost always help?

Why is it that we lose that awe when we see other people? The experience of seeing a new born baby, love at first sight, or seeing a loved one after being gone for a while, are often different from seeing anyone else. Why?

Is it that a new born baby isn't trying to sell us anything, or make us do anything? Or that only in some magical love at first sight do we actually want to buy whatever they're selling or do whatever they want us to do?

I have a hard time believing it is that simple. I think it might have something to do, with that babies, love at first sight, or loved ones we haven't seen in a while, are three groups of people we don't already have something new we want them to do or be, we are more interested in who they already are, and what they do. It is easy to see someone, and within a matter of seconds think of something we would rather them be or do. It seems at times we don't even notice people unless they are doing something we think they shouldn't do.

I've never heard someone say, "Wow, what an awesomely ordinary person, in beautifully normal situation!" It sounds odd, and even sort of cruel, although, what is more odd is all of us frantically trying to prove we are extraordinary, and not caring how we prove it. It is passion that will carry us to do extraordinary things, not the fear or being ordinary.

I raced motorcycles throughout high school and through part of college. I preferred just riding instead of racing, although

I did race quite a bit. Some of the obstacles posed risks that were too risky to enjoy at race speed. As I improved, at that new faster speed, more of the obstacles became too risky to enjoy. A friend I raced with commented the same sentiment, and I asked why he raced more than I did. He said it was the only thing he was good at. He was good, but he also started when he was three years old, and had a head start on people like me who didn't start till I was twelve. I realized that starting so early, he doesn't ever remember not being extraordinary at it. It likely seemed like a magic ticket to avoiding the dreadful feeling of ordinariness to him.

I don't know what his dossier of injuries would look like, but probably similar to mine. I broke both of my legs in one dirt biking accident, broke my wrist and arm in another, and knocked myself out in various other accidents. Though there are parts of it I miss, I don't feel obligated to keep riding. I haven't really ridden since before medical school, and my friend is still does.

It is odd that feeling average or below average is often scarier than breaking both our legs.

Shame is the idea that only extraordinary people are worth connecting to, and only extraordinary actions are worth recognizing. This idea distorts the way we see things, that something like riding a dirt bike stops being what it is, which is an instrument of kinetic art, and becomes only the desperate and dangerous means for avoiding shame. Shame reduces everything to being either the means to avoid shame or the means that shame is being put on us.

If we let it, shame tells us that friendship is just the means to avoid shame by proving we are worth connecting to. Shame also tells us the opposite, that being open with someone is just ammunition for shame to be thrown on us later.

In introducing a map of the mind and emotion, it was necessary to lay a foundation, because the fundamental basis the map derives its usefulness from seems counterintuitive.

To be loved, we must love first, and to love first, we must love ourself, but to love ourselves we must try to love others first. It turns out, our failed first attempt to love, was really the only possible beginning of love. Like a baby learning to walk, any step no matter how awkward or unsuccessful is the first step towards walking. We've already started loving, and we are probably closer to doing it well than we think.

Love is seeing an asset to life and supporting it. We can't pick and choose what assets we want to see or recognize. This doesn't mean whatever asset we happen to stumble into, that we have to invest all of our energy in it—it means simply that we allow ourselves to see assets where ever they are. Where we choice to invest our time and energy is up to us.

There is a part of our mind that sees assets, and there is no use in trying to turn that part of us off when looking at certain people we don't want to see value in, and turn it back on when looking at other people we do want to see value in. There is another part of our mind that sees logic, or risks, and a third part of our mind that weighs the assets and the risks and actually chooses to invest time and energy into. There are many ways we could label them, but one is by their type of function. The three functions are the artist, the engineer, and executive. The artist sees what assets could be added to, the engineer sees what risks could be subtracted from, and the executive chooses how to do it.

The artist function, (Intuition) and Engineer function, (intellect) are somewhat opposing functions. Like the difference between linear and non-linear thinking, quantity or quality, sensitive or specific, inclusive or exclusive, chronological or non-chronological, equity or partisan, non-critical or critical. The artist function is the process of linearly collecting all possible assets to invest in. The executive function is the process of then sorting through it all the assets and correlating the associated risks. The executive function then takes all of that information and makes a decision.

To find value, we have to assume there is value everywhere, and then compare, contrast and differentiate them. Then to find more value, we have to once again assume there is value everywhere, and then compare, contrast and differentiate them again, but this time more efficiently, because we have the results of our last value assessment to use as a standard for comparison.

Using a specific example of art, writing, and its associated engineering counterpart, editing:

I have heard many people say they are "Grammar Police," and that they read a lot, and notice all the mistakes, and want to fix them. On the other hand, I have heard many people who like writing say, that editing is a soul grinding experience. I am in the later camp, I like to write, but out of necessity have started developing my editor or "literary engineer" function to edit out the mistakes.

The cycle of writing and editing can happen many times for the same book. This book for example was completely rewritten from scratch five times over more than a decade. I have found that not only the same book improves as it is edited or rewritten, but each thing I write and edit, increases my ability to write and edit for the next project.

We were not born either an artist, an engineer or an executive, and whether we realize it or not, despite which one overall we identify with most, in every situation we are supposed to use each. Where conflict arises is when we assume a situation is a job for just one role, and someone else thinks it's a situation for a different role.

For example, a common conflict might arise if one person assuming the artist role is focused on what they would like added, which would be empathy and understanding from the other person concerning a difficult situation they are in. Meanwhile the other person assuming the engineer role could be focused on what should be subtracted, which is the problem from the situation, and try to fix it.

Since the artist function can only add, and the engineering function can only subtract, it is the executive function that must take the best of each and take the best parts of each and work them together. It takes some practice to use the executive function to see both sides, instead of splitting off to one side or the other. Our executive function must become more than just a mere critic, by having allowing it to sort through both the ideas from artist and engineer functions.

If we look at a situation as an artist, and then take the best ten percent of what we think we should add, and then look at it as an engineer and subtract the top ten percent biggest risks, it will be a lot easier for our executive function to connect the two.

Chapter 5

A.A. Milne in Winnie-the-Pooh said, "You can't stay in your corner of the Forest waiting for others to come to you. You have to go to them sometimes."

Why not explore the whole forest—It doesn't mean we have to live in the same part of the forest as someone else, but see that there was something that makes it worth living there for someone.

Something that has helped me, is I have made it a game is to figure out why someone else likes what they like. The game of life for me has changed from trying to avoid shame, to trying to find what someone enjoys.

After I can genuinely see where some's interest in something comes, I feel more able to conclude what I think about it. It doesn't mean I have to play along to figure it out, although sometimes it helps—It means I save my critique till after my analysis.

I raced motorcycles, and I wouldn't want anyone feeling obligated to spend a lot of money to go out and break their legs in order to enjoy what I enjoy, but someone should be able to see me flying through the air without wings, and dancing through the uneven terrain to the music of the engine taunting the ground, and see where the enjoyment comes from.

When one person sees something as an artist, and someone else sees it as an engineer, the resulting conflict is not because either are trying to be mean, they just aren't seeing the whole picture. If this difference in approach isn't noticed and understood, we might assume someone has devilish motives when their motives are really just vague or immature. Even if we first assess assets to add to, then risks to take away, our plan still might come to attempting to resolve a problem mostly by adding, while another person going through the same process sees the best plan as mainly subtracting risks. This often has more to do with each person's past experience than how much they want to annoy another person, even though that's not how it feels.

To quote Gary Chapman, author of The Five Love Languages, "People tend to criticize their spouse most loudly in the area where they themselves have the deepest emotional need." I would amend it to say, "we tend to conflict with people in the area of our greatest emotional or intellectual immaturity.

The less mature the need more infantile the ability to fill that need is. It is no wonder that a need with someone feels mostly helpless and completely dependent on others for the

fulfilment of that need would have such temperamental
behavior. Seeing a conflict with a person from that point of view
makes it more understandable.

Just as it doesn't make sense that a baby would cry
because they are tired instead of being quiet and going to sleep,
it doesn't make sense that people criticize and blame in things
they are immature in. Sometimes it doesn't seem someone is
immature in something because they seem to know a lot about
it, but knowing how to criticize about something or find a
rationale to blame is not the same as knowing how to do
something.

A baby either plays with food or actually eats it. What
does an adult do? We can either eat it, throw it away, put it in
the refrigerator for later, give it to someone else still play with it
if we want. It is a lot easier to make better decisions when we
see more possibilities.

Why is it that we are born not knowing whether olives
are food or a toy to play with? Because it is not either, an olive
is an olive. It is eatable and can be entertaining. In our effort to
figure out what things are we have to make assumptions. As we
start to understand things better, our assumptions of things
become closer to the reality of what they are.

We only find out that our assumption is not accurate
when an expectation we build with that assumption fails—this
challenges our assumption, and forces us to remake the
assumption with the new information. Often our assumptions are
challenged not because we purposely tested them, but because
we crashed into something. What we choose to test and what we
notice we are crashing into determines the order we learn
things—we all learn things in a different order.

When a baby throws all their food on the floor and then
cries for more, we don't get mad and tell them they had their
chance, we just give the baby more food. We should understand
that although in some aspects of our life we are definitely an
adult, in some aspects of our life we are all definitely children,
and that's okay, there's still time to keep growing.

There are a lot of things in life to figure out. If we start
on different ends of the list of things as someone else, the world
will seem quite a bit different as we each discover different parts
first. How will we know what all is good until we have really
experienced it all?

What we find all too often is really just what has found
us. Growing up, we only know the food served to us. A friend
from Mexico was stunned when visiting Paraguay because he

could not find a bottle of hot sauce anywhere. I had a similar experience in Mexico where I struggled to find any chocolate that didn't have red pepper powder in it.

Music in America predominately is in half tones, where one octave contains twelve notes, however in other parts of the world they predominately have music in quarter tones, doubling the number of possible notes in an octave. Quarter tones sound very odd to me having grown accustomed to very clear and distinct harmonies, but I'm sure to someone accustomed to quarter tones, they would find the harmonies from half tones bland or empty. What we look for is what we have been taught to look for, so much so, that we don't realize how much we are not seeing or enjoying.

I have three monitors for my computer, yes, that sounds over the top, but the reason I bring that up, is my nieces and nephews were over, and wanted to watch a video. After I started the video another suggested a different video, and I ask them what we should do, and they said watch both. That seemed odd to me, but I did it, then another suggested a third video. There we were, watching three videos at once; it was too much chaos for me to focus on anything. I was surprised to see that it didn't bother any of the four children at all. Each would watch one and then randomly switch to another. I realized that I was taught not to talk when someone else was talking, and that loud things were annoying. I guess I was inadvertently looking for what was or wasn't annoying, and not for what actually was. My nieces and nephews who had not learned this bias were looking for something else, and finding it.

We are not born knowing what a mess is, what is yucky, or what's annoying, but those all too often seem to be the focus of conversation with children, and then we wonder why most of what we see seems yucky, a mess or annoying. This is part of the reason our self-talk or internal-narration is so depressing.

This isn't to say that there aren't messes, or things that are yucky—it means that our perception is biased by what we already know to look for... until we make a serious effort to figure out what we don't know that we don't know. If we don't explore what we don't know to look for, it will be like grocery shopping with only the intention of replacing what was previously bought, and never exploring things we don't know we would love if we considered them.

What we happen to find determines what we know. What we know is what we look for, and what we look for is what we are most likely to see. This cycle influences the options we see, which limits our possible actions, which limits what value we see.

The preferences and convictions we have are the ones we stumbled into, and they might change at least a little when we see them in context with everything else we have yet to see. It is hard to imagine anything changing our preferences or convictions, but it is impossible to imagine what we don't know we don't know yet.

I have found that if someone else's preferences or convictions seem to clash with mine, that I or both of us is going to learn something, and so I try to focus on what new value I will find, instead only dreading how inconvenient it might be.

We all have a lot more in common that is immediately apparent. It is difficult, especially in the heat of the moment when someone seems to be opposing us, to try to find what value or logic they are presenting that might be new, but as long as we don't get triggered and reflexively react, we probably will find something good.

For example, in the process of writing this book, someone before even reading it, just hearing me explain a few concepts said, "You need some quotes so that people know you are not just making this stuff up..." I was triggered, especially since they hadn't even read my book yet. Despite not wanting to validate the comment by thinking about it, I did. Then when another person gave some feedback about a part they didn't understand, a few quotes came to mind that reinforced that idea well. It wasn't long before one quote turned to two, and then I rewrote the whole first half of the book after realizing that it did lay a good foundation, a necessary foundation for seeming several new ideas.

The seemly unwarranted statement went further, I realized a whole side of my journey to figure out connection that was very real, but that I was unaware of. The comment to add quotes hurt because I felt books had let me down. That seems like a big generalization to blame all books, but as a kid I had no idea how much of a generalization that was, plus it was sub-conscious, so I didn't know I had made it till I was offended by books being praised.

I felt like I was forced to make the journey to understand life and connection on my own, that besides some inspiration is survival books like Hatchet or My Side of the Mountain, that books, movies and school has only taught me how to barely survive. The only books that really helped me on my journey while I was in it instead of just validating things I had to learn myself, were those of C.S. Lewis, and I didn't want readers to think he was my only resource. I had read a lot of books and found a lot of useful things in them, but felt like it was only once I had found the answer myself that I could see it in other people's writing. Once that happened, I started seeing what I had found everywhere, and not in a conformation bias sort of way.

I realized that the comment to add quotes hit me so hard, because I was trying to prove something, that I didn't need all those books that only seemed to help once I didn't need help anymore. I realized that the resentment went pretty deep, so deep that on the surface it looked like something completely different than what it was at the core. I realized that I thought I was asking for advice when really I just wanted validation. My hurt feelings had almost nothing to do with my book, and just about everything to do with my ego.

Even now, I am inserting this passage because of a comment of someone who read it. I thought the book was done, and slightly frustrated I am still here adding more, am realizing that the obsession to be able to check off a box, to feel done, is pervasive and strong. Yes, this book does have to be published at some point, but if I would have rushed it, I would not feel the way I do right now in this moment. I wouldn't wholly feel that it's okay to admit our mistakes and petty resentments no matter how silly and self-absorbed they seem.

Life doesn't come with an instruction manual, and because of that I was looking for someone to blame, instead of something to learn. Yes, maybe we have been passed down some false ideas and misleading implications. For example, why five out of the seven emotions in English don't even have a positive way to describe them, and that of the two emotions which have positive connotations, one doesn't have a negative way to say it, when all seven are really neutral.

Yes, it would have been nice if someone would have sat me down and told me I wasn't broken, that emotions can be complicated, and not every thought that passes through my mind is me, but they are actually trying to do something useful. It would have been nice to know that other people felt the same as me, but since they were learning things in different orders, I would never know if it would have been better.

Yes, all that would have been great, but my sub-conscious blaming of books, peers, and society wasn't the answer. It's not that there were malicious people trying to hide the answer, there was just an absence of answer in a self-evident form. It doesn't mean people couldn't have lived happy lives till now, but the answer has been building for a long time, and I hope this is piece of the puzzle that propels us forward to an even greater era of contentment and composure, of belonging and connection.

We shouldn't be ashamed to be learning, because the only alternative to learning is ignoring, and life often throws us things we can't ignore forever. We also shouldn't be ashamed of the circumstances we were born into and the things we just happened to have learned first. Thanks to my parents I learned how to read at a very young age, but because of the books I happen to find or be assigned to read from school, I didn't like reading till halfway through college. There are many people who learn to read later than me, but learn to love reading much earlier, and that okay; we will all find all that has intrinsic value in life if we keep looking.

There is a big difference in the order we learn things, and that has a big influence on the things we know to look for, which influences what we have become sensitive to. I have found what I am most sensitive to is what I feel insecure about. If my identity about a certain thing seems at stake, I become very sensitive to evidence that suggests whether I am making progress in that area or not.

I have found that if I get triggered, it is a good indicator that there is something I identify as having that I still need to work on. If Gary Chapman, author of The Five Love Languages is right, that people criticize most where they have the biggest emotional need, and if I am right, that we are most sensitive to what we are most immature in, then that means when we get triggered, we actually have something very specific in common with the person who offended us...

Different than when someone gives advice, when someone criticizes us and we take it personally, it just means that we are both competing to have the same identity but approaching it from opposite directions. This means we will learn better what we were trying to prove by seeing the opposite half of it the other person sees.

All too often we are just reacting to what we are sensitive to instead of acting for ourselves, and doing what we actually want to do. Knowing we are sensitive to what we just happened to stumble into, means we spend a lot of time not being ourselves. In fact, if we regard who we are by our preferences and convictions, we won't even know ourselves until we see the big picture of life completely and see everything in context in order to properly choose a preference and conviction.

We have the ability to be more than the sum of our past circumstances and present obstacles, that is, if we are willing to look at why we react to things instead of just getting triggered.

If what we stumbled into was the feeling of being rejected, abandoned, taken advantage of, unappreciated, or deceived, we will likely overcompensate, and be hyper vigilant to make sure it doesn't happen again. If rejection was what we stumbled into for example, we might be looking intensely to see if there is any barely detectable rejection when in reality a situation has very little to do with acceptance or rejection. While we may be hyper sensitive or reactive to rejection, someone else might be the same way with being deceived, which means we will experience the same situations very differently.

If we let them, our festering wounds will steer our life more than our growing convictions. It may take longer to find deep convictions if we are fixated on avoiding pain instead of finding something worth enduring pain for. Running away from where we think we want to be least is different than running towards where we want to be most.

It is easy to get so distracted running from what we don't want, that we can't focus on the things we have found worth running to. This is probably why we get so excited when someone shares a conviction with us, because that means that someone else is running towards the same thing as us, which helps us focus on it instead of being scared about what people will think. Having someone validate what we see worth in helps us gain some certainty in our direction by not second guess ourselves so much.

C.S. Lewis said, "Friendship is born at that moment when one person says to another: 'What? You, too? I thought I was the only one.'"

Friendship is born when there is something in the two separate worlds of perspective that us and someone else live in gain in common and can be shared. Since we all actually live in the same world, everything should be common, and will be in common once our perspective gets close enough to objective reality.

Chapter 6

I have found there are four bridges over pitfalls we must cross on our own before we can truly connect with someone else. It is convenient, that our ability to connect is not dependent with whether the other person can or wants to cross those bridges themselves... although obviously it will be a deeper if they do.

Each situation has many components, and each one we either already have an assumption about or will have to make one. These assumptions will be close enough to objective reality that we will be able to see what someone else sees if we build bridges over the four common pitfalls of perception while making an assumption.

The four pitfalls we must build bridges to cross in each situation are:

1) Entertaining impossibilities
2) Distortion from ego-centricity
3) Bias towards what we think we can control
4) Infatuation with sensations, and personification of ideas

These four pitfalls are distortions in cognition, perspective, perception, and feeling. Each bridge we build leads us into a new stage of awareness, and with that improved awareness the assumption more closely matches what it really is.

Each situation in life is a new experience, and these four bridges must be built and then crossed each time. Some situations will be similar to ones we have already been in, and we will be able to build and cross the bridges faster each time. As we get more competent using all the interpersonal tools, the bridge building will be a smooth and quick process. If there is one tool we avoid using for whatever reason, when it is the tool required for a certain bridge, we get lost trying to find another way around.

The reason some things seem to come more naturally to us, is because we just happened to have the opportunity to develop the needed tool for that situation. We shouldn't restrict ourselves to what we just happen to be good at now. If we use the right tool for the job, and approach each experience as it comes to us to the best of our ability, we will become proficient with all of them, and nothing will stop us from seeing the big picture of life.

If we don't use the correct interpersonal tool, what we do will be counterproductive, and because of the negative ramifications I will call it an interpersonal weapon.

There are three types of tool or weapons, those that are intuitive based, will-power based, and intellectually based. These are not tools or weapons certain types of people use, but tools or weapons that come from different systems of our psyche: the artist function, the engineering function and the executive function.

When approached with a situation, we could look through this list and see which tool would probably work the best. Or if we have had a conflict, we could look at the list of weapons and see which weapon we used, and what tool we should replace it with.

The intuitive based tools are:
1) Fairness, 2) Forgiveness, 3) Open-mindedness, 4) Kindness, 5) Enthusiasm, 6) Compassion, and 7) Appreciation.

The will-power based tools are:
1) Teamwork, 2) Prudence, 3) Curiosity, 4) Love, 5) Perseverance, 6) Acceptance, and 7) Hope.

The intellectual based tools are:
1) Leadership, 2) Humility, 3) Creativity, 4) Social intelligence, 5) Honesty, 6) Investigation, and 7) Humor.

The intuitive weapons are:
1) Exploitation, 2) Obligation, 3) Intolerance, 4) Pseudo-altruism, 5) Rage, 6) Provoke pity, and 7) Complaining.

The will-power based weapons are:
1) Leeching, 2) Fanaticism, 3) Pride, 4) Bartering, 5) Relentlessness, 6) Competitiveness, and 7) Skepticism.

The intellectual based weapons are:
1) Manipulation, 2) Intrusiveness, 3) Uncreativity, 4) Exclusion, 5) Deceit, 6) Ego inflation, and 7) Dogmatization.

Interpersonal tools take practice to be able to use and get positive or productive results. For example, I'm sure we have told the truth at some point and regretted the hassle it created or hurt it caused to someone else. Or times we tried to be a leader and had it not work out like we would have hoped. There are also times we told a lie and seemed to avoid a lot of hassle and heartache because of it. Also, maybe there have been times we just let the team carry us instead of trying to be a leader and it seemed to prevent a lot less stress. There are reasons we have our preferred set of tools that we use for just about everything. There are also reasons why we have a set of weapons we use for situations where nothing else seems to work.

If we don't have a tool or even a weapon we know we can competently use for a situation, we can't respond to the situation, and it just happens to us. This is the first stage of awareness: Victim mentality. If we were asked why we were doing something, we would have no rationale, or might not even be aware we were doing something. This is because we don't see any way to interact with our situation, so what we do in the victim stage has nothing to do with the actual situation at hand.

The five stages of awareness are:

1) Victim Mentality
2) Fighter mentality
3) Creator mentality
4) Co-Creator mentality
5) Unadulterated Life or The Big Picture.

1) **Victim Mentality**: We all have to start at victim mentality for each assumption we make, because before we know what something is, we don't know, and we are helpless to do anything, until we know enough in order to figure out what we possibly could do. That seems obvious, but how often does life surprise us, and we get mad at ourselves for not knowing, but how could we know until we find out? The first thing we find in a situation is the most poignant thing about it, pain.

The only thing we see in situation in victim mentality is pain—not pain that is the associated cost of some asset, just straight pain. This means that the only way to escape the pain has nothing to do with the source of the pain, and that is to just distract ourselves from it. The hallmark of this stage of awareness is that it is chalked full of emotionally charged language. Instead of making the situation better changing something about the situation, we change the way we talk about it. This is in hope that someone who has control in the situation will hear our cry and change the situation for us. That person who potentially has control to change our situation is... us, but we don't believe there is anything we can do, because of our assumption that our previous efforts were all we could do and weren't enough. "I tried *everything* already and it didn't work at *all*," is the biggest obstacle in this stage.

The reason we feel we have tried everything and it hasn't worked, is because we wanted something from a situation that was impossible. This is because we aren't aware of ourselves as being part of the situation, especially being one of the only parts of a situation we can change. In the victim mentality stage we attempt to change people and the nature of things.

"I want this to be what it's not!" would be the accurate way to describe it. "I want to eat ice cream and not exercise and lose weight and feel healthy..." We can't change the relationship between diet, exercise and health, but we can change our relationship to diet and food, and thereby change our relationship to health. Doing anything the first time is often difficult, and it is true, we have likely tried and failed, but we failed because we set up the impossible to do. It is not a waste, what happens when we fail helps us identify what we are actually trying to do.

The hallmark feeling of this stage of awareness is shame. We don't see our relationship to what might be causing the shame, just the symptoms of it. We have control over our reaction to shame, and we have control over looking into what possible interpersonal duty might be contributing to the shame, but we don't have control over what people say, how they look at us, or what they think. This is one reason why shaming doesn't help someone change behavior, because the pain of the shame distracts them from the source of the pain. The focus is on the person shaming and not the possibly shameful thing they are doing. If we are doing something shameful, it's because the shameful part is too subtle for us to notice. If we want someone to see something subtle, distracting them with the poignant feeling of shame won't help.

Because this is the first stage in the journey, that means we have the least experience with the assumptions in question meaning they are least accurate and most likely to fail. Using data in a survey as an example, that information is not statistical unless there are at least thirty data points. When there are only one or two data points, the data can be easy skewed very drastically. What one or two people say can be what we assume all people are saying. Because of this, if one or two people have shamed us, we feel like everyone is shaming us.

Shame is labeling something taboo with the implication that it makes someone not worthy of connection. Because of this, in the victim stage all we see are things we shouldn't do.

We don't do anything in this stage because all we see are taboos, and it is difficult to separate them from what is not taboo, because all we know is what is what other people say is taboo which is often vague and contradicting. This is why our goals and behavior in this stage of awareness are vague and contradicting.

The lyrics to Johnny Cash's song "Hurt" show the first stage of awareness with these words, "I hurt myself today, to see if I still feel, I focus on the pain, the only thing that's real…"

1) **The first bridge** to cross which takes us from the first stage of awareness to the second is recognizing the impossibilities we are trying to entertain.

There is always something we can do in every situation, even if it is just to have patience. We might not be able to change a lot of things about a situation, and if that is the case, then patience until you see something you can do, coupled with hope that you will, are two interpersonal tools that I have found are the most appropriate tools quite often.

To leave the victim mentality stage we can start looking at possible precipitating or contributing factors to the pain in the situation we feel. If we can find even just one thing in a situation other than pain, we have moved to the next stage of awareness. "The last time I felt this way, what was similar," is a good approach.

What stops us from seeing what we can do, is being overwhelmed by the impossibilities we entertain, which feel real because they are emotionally charged, making our situation feel radically different whether we feel it is taboo or not.

We are often haunted by fears that could never happen. I'm not talking about the fear of getting struck by lightning—If you are out in a boat in a storm, the idea that you might get struck by lightening should be a serious consideration. I am talking about things that are logically impossible. For example: absolutes. "You always do that! You'll never change!" "You've never cared!" "There was nothing more I could have done!" "I will lose everything now!"

There is a tendency to emotionally charge what we say in order to get our point across. We have to ask ourselves when we find ourselves using or wanting to use emotionally charged language, "Do we think that unless we emotionally charge what we have to say to a person, they will not care to listen to us?" Or "Do we think we have to emotionally charge what we say to them, so they see value in it for themselves?"

In the first case, if the answer is yes, why are we trying to force them to listen to us? Has anyone ever successfully forced you to care about something against your will? Maybe I'm more stubborn than most, but people are typically not successful in forcing me to think a certain way if I don't want to. Surface level compliance can sometimes be forced, but not thinking or feeling.

In the second case, if the answer is yes, why do we think others are not smart enough to see the value we see on their own? And by emotionally charging something, wouldn't that just teach them to value things distorted by emotional charge? There are people that like the adrenaline that spicy food gives them so much, that food tastes bland unless it is covered in hot sauce. The same can happen with interactions, where the adrenaline associated with an emotionally charged conversation can be so addicting, that we almost completely ignore anything without it. We can't fight pain because pain is a symptom, but once we find something else beside pain, we can fight it, or fight for it. That is when we reach the second stage of awareness.

The second stage of awareness: **Fighter Mentality**, which is that there is something we can do, we don't know exactly what, but by doing several vague things there seems to be a positive effect.

For example, when someone wants to lose weight they often start several things at once, and it starts to work, but because they were all started at the same time, a few or even just could be what is helping, and the others either have no effect or are even counterproductive. Because they are all lumped together we don't know which ones to keep and which not.

It isn't as simple as just only changing one thing in our lives at a time, because some things work together. What we can do is one-by-one add them, and then once we start to see results, one by one take one away, and if there is no change, then don't worry about it, and if there is, then start doing it again.

The hallmark of the fighter stage is and "all or nothing attitude," we are either fighting so hard we can barely focus on or notice anything else. There are times in life where all we can give will be required, but those times are fairly rare. Blindly giving it all we have as fast as we can makes it difficult to see clearly what we are doing or what we should be doing.

In the fighter mentality we assume that fighting is the answer, because we feel things are directed towards us, that people and life are trying to take what we have, and that we can only keep it if we fight off life and people. For example, a rain storm doesn't particularly target you to ruin your day, it is just the result of high and low pressure and humidity. Or for example, someone that steals money, doesn't particularly want "your" money, they just want money, and circumstances may make you the target.

One big component of the fighter stage is magical thinking, in the fighter stage if we are doing ten things to fight in a situation, at least one of them is going to be completely superstitious or ridiculous, but because we see the ten as one big mass, we feel all ten are equally valid. Ironically the part based on superstition, because it is the weakest part of our action, that will be what crashes with other people. We end up fighting to defend that one ridiculous thing so much more than the other nine, that it starts to seem like the most important part. Then because we fight to defend that one ridiculous part so much, and because we are likely the only ones that believe so strongly about it, that we are singled out for it. We end up making the situation about us that originally wasn't, because we assumed that it was from the start.

In a situation, where one superstitious or ridiculous assumption we have ends up causing us so much trouble the more we try to hold onto it, that as we try to figure out how to hold on to it, we realize what it really it. If we feel like there is something we are fighting for, we should break it down into different parts, so that it is not one idea, but a concert of smaller ideas, and then find the one that is out of tune.

What brings us out of the fighter stage is making an assumption that doesn't mix in a lot of extra things that don't have anything to do with it. The goal obviously would be to have assumptions that are exactly what something is, no more and no less, but all we can do is approach that goal.

Whereas the theme of the victim stage was taboos, the theme of the fighter stage is ideals. People label us as ideal in certain ways, and it feels good to have that positive label, which is much preferable to the negative label of being taboo, but almost equally vague and contractive. Likely a young child is not literally the greatest artist in the world, but when a child draws a picture likely a label is given so far beyond their actual ability, that they will be fighting to keep that label in vain their whole life if they try to hold onto it.

The positive labels we are fighting to keep sometimes have very little to do with us, and more to do with some random compliment we got or circumstance where we felt special, that is why some of the assumptions connected with it are superstitious, because they don't exist. The question we should ask is, "Do we want to feel right, or be right?" It's not a matter of building a biased jury to prove everything, it is about actually figuring out how to do something.

It might seem scary to see the most magical parts of our assumptions striped away, but what we find when we do, it actually useful assumptions. As soon as we have one useful assumption, we now can create something.

2) **The second bridge** to cross from the Fighter stage to the Creator stage is eliminating the distortion of Ego-centricity. Because the world and all the people in it don't actually revolve around us, we start seeing the world and people for what and who they are when we see what they do actually revolve around.

After we became aware of pain in the first stage, we found something specific to fight to defend in the second stage which was the ideal parts of our self-image. After fighting we realize that not all fights are the same. After fighting everything and everyone that surrounded our pain, it is only a matter of time before we have fought everyone besides ourselves with the pain of a hurt self-image is still there. At this point we realize or are forced to realize that there are things about ourselves that we can change. We find that when we make a change something good happens, and we realize we have some control over our life, which is the third stage.

"When we are no longer able to change a situation, we are challenged to change ourselves." — Viktor E. Frankl, Man's Search for Meaning

In a situation, once we realize there is something we can do that we know directly is related to what we want to do, then we can use it and create something.

The third stage of awareness is the "**creator stage.**" In this stage we have at least connected wanting to doing for at least for one thing.

In driving a car, once we learn we can turn left, that means we don't have to just go straight, but it also means that until we learn we can also turn right, that we will be going most places the long way.

Whereas the big picture of life appeared vague and contradictive in the victim and fighter stage, in the creator stage, we at least clearly see one part of the big picture.

We quickly realize that our ability to create is only in controlled situations, and realize the determining factor in whether we can create something or not, dependents on who and what is around us. We then learn to avoid places or people that we don't feel we can control. Whereas we feel we are controlling life, really, we are just relegating ourselves to that small portion of life that we feel we can control. In this stage what we think we like and what we choose to do, has to do with whether we feel we can control it or not.

At this stage we can only create certain things from what we have stumbled into through our fighting. If someone else has stumbled into the same things, and sees those things in the same way, friendship can be made through that common interest. This tempts us to look for people who share our common interest instead of trying to see something the way someone else sees what they enjoy.

It's not that we are oblivious in this stage, but we often get so fixated on trying to figure out if the factors in a situation can be altered so that it can be the situation that we need in order to create. We get distracted by trying to figure out if things supports what we want to create, or how something can be used for that purpose, that we don't get a good look at what things actually are.

In this stage there is a tendency to only see value in people that share the same narrow understanding as us, and see value in things that are useful for what we want to do.

3) **The third bridge** to cross is recognizing bias towards wanting only what we think we can control. It's okay to be in a situation we are not in complete control of. By avoiding situations we can't control, we just end up isolating ourselves from experiences which would help us learn how to create in other situations.

The more we learn about the specific thing we figured out how to create, the more we realize that very few people share our exact common purpose, because it has become so particular. We then come to the conclusion that either everyone else is crazy/incompetent, or others have very refined but particular things they have figured out how to create. This usually doesn't happen because we consider the question, like the other two stages, it eventually crashes its way into our awareness.

Just as we moved into the fighter stage from the victim stage by looking for what surrounded pain, likewise we move from the creator stage to the co-creator stage when we start to look around what we create. We start from that one portion of the big picture of life we see clearly, and explore what surrounds it till it all comes into focus.

The fourth stage of awareness is the **co-creator stage**. At this stage we see the big picture of life enough to be able to create whatever we want. If we can create anything, then we also can relate to whatever anyone else wants to create. Although, just because we see a way to make whatever we want, doesn't mean we know the best way to do it. Some things will be harder to create and that might make them seem not worth it. In this stage we see the big picture, but there are still parts of the picture that seem to have more color, more excitement, and more nostalgia. We still spend more time in one part than another, and so some parts of the picture though fairly clear, are still unfamiliar.

Just because we know how to use something, doesn't mean we like it. For example, the ocean, I know how to swim, I know how to operate a boat, and I even know how to scuba dive, and I enjoy them, but I still see the ocean as principally a dangerous thing.

I think my suspicion of the ocean is mostly because I am unfamiliar with it, that is why I learned how to scuba dive. The first time I went below the surface with my scuba gear I couldn't control my breathing, I was breathing super-fast and deep. I know how bad hyper-ventilating is, and feeling like a fairly self-disciplined person, I was frustrated that I couldn't control myself. I was aware instruments I was using, and of the possible creatures I would see diving, and the risks, but still I was much more comfortable on land than in the sea. Combined with the excitement of seeing a sea horse, and all sorts of fish, was the fear I felt, which made it difficult to appreciate fully what I was really seeing.

It was two dives before I could somewhat control my breathing, and about five before I felt I could breathe normally. Knowing how to scuba dive didn't mean I could do it well, that took experience. In unfamiliarity there are certain sensations that we have to not let trigger us so that we can actually focus on where we are and what we are doing instead of how unfamiliar the circumstance is.

It makes it more difficult to see what someone else is seeing, when we are factoring in sensations and factors that the other person doesn't have. The scuba instructor was more comfortable in the ocean than on land. Whereas there were things on land I could handle like the drama of life, but figured that the ocean would get me, for him it proved the opposite. The goal is to be okay with wherever we are.

In Madeleine L'Engle's book A Wrinkle in Time, the main character Meg is on a journey to find her father, who has traveled across the universe. Assumptions about life between a forty-year-old man and a twelve-year-old girl are probably equivalent to different sides of the universe, but she travels it through the idea of a tesseract. A tesseract is a four-dimensional cube where all the sides are equal. If each side of a cube is the longer or shorter depending on how familiar we are with it, they it won't be a cube unless we familiar with everything.

In neuroscience there is a concept called plasticity, which means that neuro-circuits that are used and the outcome is rewarded get strengthened, making them faster. If there are twenty-one interpersonal tools, and the neuro-pathways to one particular tool are much faster than the others, that will create some bias. The idea of the tesseract is having the neuro-pathways to all twenty-one interpersonal tools equally as fast.

For me, seeing how someone could live in the ocean most their life is hard to relate to, but that is because I am trying to imagine myself doing, and not imagining it for what it is.

If a flower blooms in the forest where there is no one there to see it, does it still have color? Is it still beautiful? Yes, things are what they are, and personifying them into being more or less than they are, is a way of valuing or devaluing something for some reason other than what it actually is. When no measurement is exaggerated or minimized, when each length of each side of this cube of life is equal which it should be, we can find someone even if they are across the universe from us. This doesn't mean that we have to live at the bottom of the sea, but when circumstance takes us there, and if the only hesitation we have is that it is unfamiliar, then we shouldn't miss out. Scuba diving is still not the thing I want to do most if life, but I know I will have a good time if I go, especially if others there are enjoying it.

I don't identify as a scuba diver even though I went a dozen times, I don't think identifying as anything helps us connect, I think an identity just tells us how we are supposed to feel. "This isn't me, I'm not a diver," is not worth thinking if we saw value in doing it. "This is my favorite thing, I am a diver, so I have to enjoy this," is also not the right attitude either.

We would have to have a pretty odd view of other people to think something that is someone's favorite thing in life doesn't at least have five percent validity. We would also have to have a pretty odd view of ourselves to think that something we like has a hundred percent validity. What some people do may seem odd to us, but if the only reason we can think that they are doing it is because they are crazy... we are probably missing something. Things can be imprudent, or immature, but not crazy.

Is a daisy better than a dandelion? A daisy is labeled as a flower and a dandelion is labeled as a weed. They both look similar, but they can't be compared as if one is good and the other bad, they both just are what they are. They are similar in ways and different in ways, and if daisies work better for a certain reason in a certain circumstance, that great, but if we find ourselves triggered when we see a dandelion and excited when we see a daisy just because of what they are, we should ask ourselves why? A child appreciates them both, that doesn't mean we can't pull them out of our garden or lawn, but we should remember that it was blew in with the wind and grew where it was planted, we all are doing the same.

I feel like this is a difficult analogy, because I am in no way advocating for plant rights, I just think that out of all the things we could think first when seeing a dandelion, why think something negative and unproductive? Yes, there will likely be time spent to pull it up and throw it away, but if it is really the problem that you would like to fix, then wondering where it blew in from would take you to the source, and you could stop it there. In the last stage of awareness, we aren't triggered by symptoms of things, we see them for what they are, and deal directly with the source calmly and unbiasedly.

The fourth bridge to cross is Infatuation, and Personification of Ideas. We have to realize that whether or not we can sense ourself, we still exist. Whether or not we are familiar with something or not enough to be excited when we see it, doesn't mean that we shouldn't learn about it. What something does or says about our identity is irrelevant to what it is, because an identity is not real. We all see each other differently, and even if it were real, it would just be a label of our assets and risks, as if we were no more than an item to be cataloged.

There are certain things we know how to do, and which would be helpful, but we don't because of how it might look. For example, like ask for directions, accept criticism from someone younger or less titled than us, or listen to someone of an opposing political party or ideology. Even simple things like wearing a jacket when we're cold can seem difficult just because we want to control the way people see us, all in order to feel we have the self-esteem to motivate us to do what we are very capable of doing without it.

Whether or not we feel we are full of self-esteem or not, we are still capable of doing what we want, and there is no use of dreading the learning process where the enjoyment is mixed in with the apprehension of the trying.

Chapter 7

There is a debate in the psychology world whether self-esteem is a good thing.

We say that something is good or bad, but often neglect to qualify what it is good or bad for. Fatty food may be good for taste or absorption of fat soluble vitamins, and bad for avoiding metabolic syndrome, heart attacks or strokes.

C.S. Lewis writing on the nature and evolution of language said, "The truth is that words originally descriptive tend to become terms either of mere praise or of mere blame. The vocabulary of flattery and insult is continually enlarged at the expense of the vocabulary of definition. As old horses go to the knacker's yard, or old ships to the breakers, so words in their last decay go to swell the enormous list of synonyms for good and bad. And as long as most people are more anxious to express their likes and dislikes than to describe facts, this must remain a universal truth about language."

For the reason C.S. Lewis described, I will have to define self-esteem so that it can be properly considered whether it is productive or counter-productive to our pursuit of contentment and composure in life. Self-esteem is a personification of presence or absence of tiredness, the perceived ease of our circumstance or feeling of momentum. All three of these things, though possibly motivating in a way, are subjective. As much enabling motivation as absence of the sensation of tiredness or assessment of ease possibly could produce, they will also produce the same amount of disabling discouragement when they are not there.

Each time self-esteem fails us, it becomes harder to attain, because we second guess whether what feels like self-esteem is just wishful thinking. It's not that there is nothing good about self-esteem, just that it is near impossible to separate out the benefit from the harm, and not needed because there are other concrete ways of attaining motivation which are more efficient and more effective.

When confidence spontaneously appears without a logical source, it is likely that it is over-confidence. If your experience is similar to mine, over-confidence has gotten me in a lot of trouble... like two broken legs from riding my dirt bike.

The whole premise of Cognitive Behavioral Therapy is that there are distortions in thinking. We sometimes are irrational about our ability, we feel inadequate at a task despite already having done something similar that was more difficult, and ironically, we are sometimes confident in something we have almost no experience with. Yes, we might more often second-guess ourselves than not, but we likely do both be over-confident and under-confident. The way to progress beyond that, is a steady climb towards the concrete, towards objectivity, towards what's real.

Self-esteem is substituting assessment of value, for a sense of self. This means that whereas we should base our actions on whether or not we assess value, we are tempted to base our actions on whether is produces a sense of self, or self-esteem. I'm probably not the only one who while at a swimming pool wanted to feel that everyone else knew I was there, by doing a cannon ball and trying to make the biggest, loudest splash I could. And though I'm sure most pools in the world have been the host of many spontaneous cannonball competitions, for some reason is still is not an Olympic sport. In fact, quite the opposite, from a height of thirty-three feet, Olympic divers after many spins and twists hardly make a splash. With no accompanying noise or stray of water, it is very possible that their dive will go completely unnoticed by some people. Self esteem is the loud splash, it's hitting the water knowing everyone will feel or at least hear the wave you make.

Self-esteem is a subjective thing, and if we let it govern our decisions, we won't be able trust ourselves to actually do the things we find value in because of the value alone. If we feel our decisions can't be made as a result of our own judgment of value, how can we how to have results in our life that have value?

If really the case is that we don't do something because we are just tired, or distracted by something else, we have to either admit that is why we didn't do it, or lie to ourselves that maybe secretly or sub-consciously we didn't actually want to do it. It seems we would rather think we are controlled by irrational drives through our sub-conscious than feel we are so lazy that we don't do things we want to do just because we are tired. If we don't see self-esteem for what it is, something arbitrary, that is nice when it's there, but not worth chasing, then we will spend our time chasing it instead of what we want it to help us achieve. Ironically, the more we let self-esteem keep us from doing what we want, the less self-esteem we will have.

Actual momentum helps in life, and doing something simple well right before doing something harder helps us have courage or certainty, but it's just that, and nothing more—we can bounce a basketball a few times before shooting a free-throw, but we shouldn't never shoot because the ease of bouncing a ball makes us feel more comfortable.

Lasting comfort comes from finding what is concrete and building a real foundation, not from the fabricating the illusion of control, or imagination of approval. Attitude is not a fabricated emotional state we employ trick ourselves into caring enough to do something, it is posture or disposition we make towards what we want to do in spite of opposition.

What benefit would it have to let our attitude and judgment depend on how tired or hungry we are, or how hot or cold it is? This is the difference between self-esteem, and self-confidence. Self-esteem is greatly influence by temporary or false things, a fake compliment for example can be motivating, but then equally or more discouraging when we find out it was fake or mal-intended. Self-esteem is fine when it is there, but shouldn't be the goal. Self-confidence on the other hand is confidence in our ability based on honest previous experience, and it is not dependent on weather or circumstance. A pursuit towards self-esteem, will lead us to where we feel weather and circumstance will most likely be in our favor, and not where we see concrete value and logic.

Why should our excitement towards doing a thing have to do with what other people express about it? If we are authentically enjoying something and someone mockingly laughs, why should that change anything?

If someone's laugh can make the value we see in what we are doing disappear, we are letting the sensation of feeling approval or disapproval overshadow the thing itself.

Any sensation, be it excitement or similar that is not focused on an actual aspect of value or criteria of logic, will distract us and ultimately disappoint us. Positive sensations like excitement and a feeling of self-worth often accompany positive actions, but they are not the means to a life of contentment and composure or finding value and logic in life.

Whether self-esteem seems to carry us or is merely a side-effect of our effort to carry ourselves, it is often present as we cross the first three bridges. However, to cross the last bridge, we must let it go, despite how counterintuitive it may seem. It is natural to want to feel good, but it shouldn't be at the expense of doing what has value. We are told to do what feels good, but immediate gratification feels only good in the moment, and that is not enough.

Brené Brown, a researcher who has specialized in shame said about connection, "I define connection as the energy that exists between people when they feel seen, heard, and valued; when they can give and receive without judgment; and when they derive sustenance and strength from the relationship."

I believe there is an energy that is created between people even if they don't feel, seen, heard, or valued, as long as they are working towards that same goal. There is a reason why there is love and tough-love. Being a third-year medical student for example, I rarely if ever felt seen, heard or valued, but was still able to work as a team, and everyone benefited from the co-operation. Obviously, we should try to help those around us feel appreciated, but when we don't feel appreciated we shouldn't let it stop us. It's much easier if we just accept the duty to always be the one to love first, and then be pleasantly surprised when someone beats us to it.

This brings us back to the idea of attitude being a posture we assume to prepare for the obstacles that will try to prevent us from our pursuit. Self-confidence is the trust in ourselves in our capability to not be distracted by whims and weather, it's a trust in ourselves to stay focused on value and logic and not ease and comfort. This confidence is built up steadily over time. Our self-esteem comes and goes on a whim, but self-confidence is increased every time it is challenged and we prevail. It is difficult to separate the two because there is some overlap, but the point is to focus on doing what we know we should do and not worry about what we hope we feel.

A big part of self-esteem is the feeling of succeeding. Obviously, we should try our best, but the feeling of succeeding doesn't mean that we tried our best, it means that we feel we made it over the bar we set for ourselves or over the bar that someone else set for us. For example, in racing motocross, halfway through a season, I was leading a race, and I felt myself settle because I didn't want to risk the race by going faster and crashing even though I could have pushed myself a lot further. I decided I didn't care about the season overall, and I moved up a class for the next race. I found myself at the back of the leader pack, and though it pushed me more, I decided the next week to move up another class. There I was struggling to stay out of last place, but it was nice to push myself as far as I could and not worrying about season points or trophies. I got faster in the next few races in the top class than I had the rest of the season combined. Crossing the finish line in last place may not feel like succeeding, but getting back to the truck and hearing how much my lap times had improved, I knew I was succeeding. Self-confidence was the concrete trend of decreasing lap times. Self-esteem would have been contentment not pushing myself and carrying home a first-place trophy every week in a class clearly below my ability.

We should enjoy doing our best, but not settle for merely repeating our past best, we can always reflect and then do at least a little bit better. We can remember what we find, but we can't know what we are going to find before we do, and we don't have to, the surprise adds some fun to the adventure of life.

All too often we look at what we do as either successful or not—this polarization leads to us feeling as a person like a failure or a success, when in reality, with each thing we do, there is at least some part worth repeating, and some part not worth repeating.

Whether we feel like something we did was positive or not, the best thing to do would be dissect it, and see which parts of our action are worth repeating and which are not. None of our actions will be a hundred percent right, and none will be a hundred percent wrong, each action deserves a proper post-mortem.

A chemist, Roy Plunkett was doing research on refrigerants in 1945, and "failed" at storing in an air tank hundreds of pounds of tetrafluoroethylene gas for an experiment. When he went to use the gas, he turned the valve and nothing came out. Instead of throwing it out and feeling bad for failing, he cut the air canister in half. He found the inside of the air canister filled with a coating that was heat resistant, chemically inert, with such a low surface friction that most other substances would not adhere to it. He had accidently invented Teflon.

We have probably stumbled in to more greatness than we would believe, but missed it hurrying away with our head down in shame feeling clumsy and dumb.

At some point we stop chasing sensations, and start searching for what actually is, what actually has value, and what we can actually do. We start to see that there are assets and risks to everything, and it is just a matter of understanding them to know what to do, how to do it and whether it will be worth it.

We can move beyond just seeing what we know to look for. We start to see the big picture of life by trying to find what other people are looking at that we don't see. With time we start to see more, and realize even if someone else only sees a small part of the big picture, because we see the whole thing, we will know what they are talking about, and can more easily connect with them.

After crossing all four bridges for a given situation, we arrive at the final stage of awareness: **Contentment and Composure.** Once we see the big picture, and we are not controlled by mere sensations, we can calmly and unbiasedly navigate our way through life.

We will have to cross the four bridges many times, the pitfalls will be slightly different for each different thing or situation, but we get faster at building to the point it isn't very difficult. If there is a conflict, it is because we walked into the pitfall instead of crossing the bridge. The good news is that if we have come to the point that we recognize there is a conflict, and we believe there is something we can do about it besides fighting, and we are trying to change ourself instead of control someone else, in the resolution of that conflict, there is just one bridge left for us to cross. When there is something we see as black or white that is not, once we find it, we can start to see it for what it really is.

Chapter 8

Whichever of the five possible stages of awareness we are in at the moment, is all we see. When we aren't aware of something, it doesn't seem to exist to us. Anything we stumble into we weren't aware of, we just reflexively react to. Mental reflexes are life biological reflexes which are primitive, and consist of kicking, pulling away, or throwing up.

If we are talking to someone about something, we should probably figure out which stage they are in for that situation, and remember that we can only help someone move up one level of awareness at a time. If it seems like the other person is kicking or pulling away, what you are trying to communicate is at least one stage of awareness too high for them at the moment, or we don't understand something as well as we think.

It is wise to only give input when someone has a question, but it is also may be a kind thing to do, to inspire or provoke that question when it is not there yet. We need a place for new ideas, because we start off not knowing that there is something out there we should know.

In the victim stage, all we know or see is pain, and we don't know there is anything we can do about it. Pain is the easiest to see, but it doesn't have to be all we see, we just have to take the question farther beyond, "what is the pain?" and "where is it coming from?" towards, "what do I want there instead of the pain?" and "how am I going to do that?" Hunger pains are because our body wants food, and we remove the pain or avoid it by eating.

It is often we realize we don't have the answer to something before we realize we had a question about, and much before we can identify the exact question. We feel a pain in our stomach and then ask why. Life tends to do the same, we feel alone, and then we ask why. We are stopped by a problem, and then ask why. It doesn't have to be that way, we can consider questions before we need the answers.

Albert Einstein said, "It's not that I'm so smart, it's just that I stay with problems longer." He also said, "If I had an hour to solve a problem and my life depended on the solution, I would spend the first 55 minutes determining the proper question to ask... for once I know the proper question, I could solve the problem in less than five minutes."

Four good questions ask or inspire others to ask that correspond to the four bridges to connection are:

1) What impossibilities are there in what we are considering might be the cause or solution of the problem? Eg. "This pain is killing me... I would do anything to make it go away." This would be an impossibility, because pain is just a byproduct of a cause, it won't be the pain that kills us, but the cause. When we say we would do anything, it should include the idea of sitting down and figuring out what is actually going on. "This always happens to me, and always will, there is nothing I can do about it, I've already tried everything." If there really is nothing to do, why complain about it? It is unlikely that we have tried everything, and more unlikely that after actually trying to solve our problem that complaining will work where action didn't. Some things take time, and if we don't know the process to fix our problem, how would we know how long that process would take? Not knowing how long solving the problem would take, how would we know when to throw in the towel and deem it impossible?

2) What seems to be aimed at us or in reference to us? And what are the possible ways we could draw or reframe the situation not in reference to us? eg. "They did that just to make me mad!" It is impossible that someone could do something with the only motivation to make you mad. A person would have to want something else, maybe a feeling a vindication, or a feeling of self-importance, but not just for the sole purpose of making you mad. I have found most of my decisions are composed of many reasons, rarely is it just one thing. Also, we are often mostly just worried about ourselves, and so most likely whatever someone else does that may affect us, is more so about them than us. If I swam out to rescue someone drowning, and they pushed me under the water, I wouldn't assume they were just being ungrateful, or just being mean, I would assume there are in full hysterical panic and not really conscious of much of anything besides the sensation of drowning.

3) What are we trying to control? And why? It would be really convenient if we could just change everything and everyone else to fit us, but not only is that not possible, but life would seem very lifeless if everything and everyone were just our little puppets. Attempting to overcome a personal obstacle by controlling someone else, shows a discrepancy between where we are heading and where we think we will end up. It is one thing to want something, and it is a completely different thing to want something by a specific means. Eg. "I want to feel better by making them regret what they did to me." Whether or not it would be helpful to someone to regret what they did to us,

that has very little if anything to do with our happiness. I feel a sense of duty of restitution when I harm someone, but that feeling is distinctly different than the feeling when someone is trying to make me feel guilty. If someone is trying to make me feel guilty and they think that will help me or them in anyway, it makes me more sad for them considering what stress that attitude will create for them, and not how guilty I feel. We can't control the way someone feels. We can't force someone to regret something, and we can't force someone to love us, all we can do is our best to facilitate it.

4) Are we trying to actually do something we see value in, or merely just feel something? Also, where are we drawing the line to determine whether or not we feel what we wanted to feel? Eg. "I want to feel appreciated." "I want to feel understood." "If they appreciate me, they will drop everything to help me out." Or, "If they agree with everything I say, then I will know that they understand me."

In some ways life is easier with cars, hospitals and farms, but these also create new potential for accidents, malpractice and spread of infection. Like technology, ideas have been evolving, and that has created both better ways to connect, and also more barriers to connection. It was hard for me to grasp that I was not just wrestling with myself, or life, but with every bad idea with enough substance to get passed down over the last several millennia. Like bacteria evolve to become resistant to antibiotics, so too bad ideas evolve to be resistant to reason as they are passed down from one generation to the next.

Like me, I'm sure most others tried to hide their struggle with this battle we are all born into, trying to find ourselves, life and others. Now, knowing we are all going through the same thing, hopefully we don't feel we have to hide. Hopefully we don't feel we are broken or weird, we are all learning, and learning things in different orders, and that's okay.

Shel Silverstein illustrated this in a poem:

"She had blue skin,
And so did he.
He kept it hid
And so did she.
They searched for blue
Their whole life through,
Then passed right by-

And never knew."

It's okay to show our blue skin, it's okay to talk about what we find difficult in life. We think we are the only ones struggling, because hardly anyone ever talks about it, which makes it scary to talk about it. Instead of opening up, which would facilitate connection and learning, ironically we often sacrifice opportunities for connection and learning because we don't want to look broken, needy, or odd, in order to appear worth connecting to.

Mark Twain said, "It's better to keep your mouth shut and appear stupid than open it and remove all doubt." I think though we don't articulate it, this is a fear—that we are broken when we try to connection or not, but if we stay quiet about it, at least we can enjoy the benefits of appearing whole, or even at least normal.

Even if we were stupid or broken, does that mean we are unlovable? If we let the feeling that we might be broken make us feel unlovable, we will likely hide, and never find out whether or not love was possible. I know love is possible, it naturally comes out of us. Even when we feel lonely and incapable of love, that means our heart is working, just that our mind is resisting the opportunity to try. If it is an idea that is stopping us from following our heart, maybe we should discuss the idea with someone else.

Brené Brown in her book The Gifts of Imperfection said, "As much as we need and want love, we don't spend much time talking about what it means. Think about it. You might say "I love you" every day, but when's the last time you had a serious conversation with someone about the meaning of love? In this way, love is the mirror image of shame. We desperately don't want to experience shame, and we're not willing to talk about it. Yet the only way to resolve shame is to talk about it. Maybe we're afraid of topics like love and shame. Most of us like safety, certainty, and clarity. Shame and love are grounded in vulnerability and tenderness."

Worth doesn't make a connection, trust does. We have to trust ourselves, trust others, and trust that connection is possible. Listening to our heart isn't impossible, it happens intuitively, the hard part is not listening to fear.

Love is not something we must try hard to do, love comes naturally, it is trusting that love is enough—That is the hard thing to do. It sounds simple, but even when the simple answer is right in front of us, since the feeling is complicated, we often pass up the right answer to look for a complicated answer to match it.

In the 1300s somewhere between seventy-five and two-hundred million people died from the black plague, which was a bacteria carried by fleas. Fleas are not a new problem, and the cure has been widely known long before the 1300s. It was simply to shave your hair off, wear clothes made from something coarse like goat hair, and to cover your skin in ash. The fleas lay eggs that stick to our hair, and with the hair gone, there is nowhere for the eggs to stick. The ash has the chemical hydroxide, which is enough to make the skin unlivable for the fleas.

Everyone knew that anyone with a shaved head and ash on their skin meant that they knew they had fleas. To avoid the shame, many people would rather put up with the fleas, as long as other people didn't think they had them. Maybe the quote before Mark Twain coined his was, "It's better to keep your hair and appear free from fleas than shave your head and remove all doubt."

Besides itching and inflammation, fleas were fine... sort of... that is, until those fleas got infected with the plague, and spread that deadly infection. Instead of shaving their heads, people tried any other thing, and about half of Europe died.

We shouldn't be embarrassed to be human, and we shouldn't feel stupid that we're embarrassed, we should just talk about it, and get over it. Feeling unworthy of connection just for being human is the emotional plague, and we won't know what it means to be human until we talk to other humans and realize they are scared and confused and definitely not perfect either.

Chapter 9

Benjamin Franklin once said, "We are all born ignorant, but one must work hard to remain stupid."

Ignorant comes from the word to ignore. Naïve comes from the root of the word nativity, it means born. We do ignore things, but that is because we are naïve—if we really knew something was important, we wouldn't ignore it, we may get distracted and forget about it, but that is different. We don't know what we don't know, and we don't know how important the things we don't know are, because we don't know what they are.

We grow up as we stop wanting things to be what they are not. We grow when we want to figure out what things actually are. We can replace the fear of change, we the excitement for understanding. Ignorance isn't bliss; dreaming we are eating doesn't fill our belly, and dreaming we are content with life is not the same as it really happening.

My experience has been that I am always learning, sometimes the hard way and sometime the easy way. The hard way is resisting change in our naïve picture of life until the pressure of reality finally breaks it. We learn the easy way by accepting the possibility of change and looking for what is real wherever we can. Learning from others by watching their mistakes or listening to their insights has helped learn more things the easier way than I would have otherwise. We need to allow room for new ideas when they come. Something about, "A work in progress," just doesn't seem appealing, we want to be a finished product, but being a finished product means we won't experience any greater contentment or composure in life than we already have.

We are often proud about what we know and ashamed of what we don't know, but pride of what we already know doesn't encourage us to learn more, and feeling ashamed of what we don't know doesn't motivate us either. We should be excited to find out what we don't know, not just so what we want to do is not undermined by unforeseen details, but that we can find all life has to offer.

A person's popularity and self-esteem will go up and down randomly, but learning and growing can happen at a steady pace as life gives us opportunities to ask new questions and find new answers every day. What we do with what we learn to make things better is up to us, and makes all the difference in what we get out of life. If obstacles in life are inevitable, then we might as well make it a game and enjoy the challenge, because seeing obstacles as a prison won't motivate us to do anything productive about it.

In 1898 Marie Curie discovered the chemical element Radium, which is radioactive. This gave it an interesting glow, and by 1910, was put in food products, make-up, glow in the dark watches, and many other products, some claiming to be medical devices. It wasn't until 1925, after a full factory full of workers had gotten very sick, and all eventually died prematurely, that radium was pulled from consumer markets. Sometimes we are working but our effort is counterproductive, because the understanding it was based on is wrong. Ideas can be dangerous.

Like Franklin said, though we are born ignorant, we won't remain that way unless we work against the natural learning process. Just like the workers painting radium on watch dials, we have all been born in a complex world, with some ideas we don't realize are destroying us from the inside out. It would have been worse if the danger of Radium was ignored and people kept dying. We can't avoid all danger in life, but when we do something, we can reflect on how it actually turned out compared to how we thought it would, and remember what we find. The consequence of our actions is not always readily apparent, but avoiding ever finding out what an action does, is dangerous, no matter how nostalgic or innocent the idea may seem.

When we plan to do something, we should plan a way to see if it does what we want it to do and any other unintended consequences it may have.

Advertisers use slogans, because they know that is all we are likely to remember, and it will be enough to get us to buy their product. While this may be enough to make a decision on which everyday item to buy where the competitors version likely is almost identical anyways, it isn't enough to make real life choices. Many popular quotes recorded throughout history, especially out of the context they were said, and isolated down to one or two simple sentences, makes them very susceptible to misinterpretation. Though a quote can feel like a well thought idea, catchy or not, it can't replace our own judgement. Every thought starts with one sentence, and what memorable phrases we heard growing up often have a greater chance of being that first sentence than an idea completely our own. When we go down the same set of roads our collection of idioms sends us, we will end up in the same places, and not realize it was the context they gave that lead us to the conclusions we made, not our out real thoughts or feelings.

An example of a phrase that could be interpreted many different ways: Charles Darwin said, "A man's friendships are one of the best measures of his worth."

If it is meant that if you trust someone, you will likely trust their close friends, or that the more we learn how to love, the easier and quicker we make friends, then it is useful. If it is interpreted, that someone is allowed to have a sense of self-worth and feel good about themselves if they have many friends, or anything even remotely similar, I think it could be damaging.

It is interesting how we claim our feelings as our own, but often leave them in the control of other people. This happens when we confuse or combine our authentic emotions with our sense of self-worth or feeling of self-esteem. Until we are able to separate them, we have to be okay with them being mixed.

Ambivalence means to hold more than one feeling at a time. How does it feel when we admit to someone that we were wrong? Probably mixed feelings. There is the feeling of confidence that we can do hard things, the feeling that there was justice in being honest about it, and wisdom in recognizing mistakes. There is also probably the uneasy feeling of vulnerability, the feeling of insignificance, and the feeling of embarrassment. Ambivalence means accepting that all of those thoughts and feeling can coexist. Sanity means recognizing that some thoughts and feelings are objective and useful, and others are not, and poise is understanding that separating them out may take some time... and that's okay.

When there is a big influx of mixed feelings, we often feel too overwhelmed to separate and challenge them. At times we entertain completely opposite ideas or feelings, which is fine for it to start that way, but not stay that way. For example, think that something we did was the smart thing to do, but still feel stupid for doing it. For exampling, feeling dumb for asking for help. Asking for help is a smart thing to do, there is nothing dumb about it, so although that feeling may tag along, we should know that it is invalid.

Psychologist Otto Rank said, "For the only therapy is life. The patient must learn to live, to live with his split, his conflict, his ambivalence, which no therapy can take away, for if it could, it would take with it the actual spring of life."

We are always doing our best. Like the power in our house, it is almost always running at a hundred and-twenty volts, the difference is what we choose to plug into it. We are thinking and feeling at a hundred percent at all times; there are times we can think of a better way we could have used that energy, but just because we can think of something better later, doesn't mean we were purposely trying to think bad or purposely being negligent. In making a decision, it's not possible to weigh out the options, and then not pick the best one. Yes, it is very possible that something we've weighed into the equation was very impractical, but if the idea would have worked or been true, it would have been the best decision.

Hanging on each side of the balance of choice, is often many different reasons supporting each side, each reason containing a different level of confidence. Yes, letting something weigh in with only five percent confidence against something with ninety percent confidence is often imprudent, but in the cases where something with five percent confidence behind it has worked out, it has been quite the discovery. Yes, we often feel stupid for taking such impractical risks, but we are not alone in seeing the value in taking risks.

Helen Keller said in her book, The Open Door, "Life is either a daring adventure or nothing at all."

Neil Gaiman said in, The Graveyard Book, "If you dare nothing, then when the day is over, nothing is all you will have gained."

Ralph Waldo Emerson said, "Don't be too timid and squeamish about your actions. All life is an experiment. The more experiments you make the better."

Mark Twain, "Why not go out on a limb? That's where the fruit is."

It is easy in life to become more scared of ridicule from others than stagnancy in our personal growth. Life is not a menagerie, and it won't be worth more later because it's still in its original box.

"The only real mistake is the one from which we learn nothing." — Henry Ford

We often get distracted figuring out what to do with the feeling of failure, instead of considering the positive implications of what we just learned. Any single thing we learn, should change everything else we know for the better—everything real is part of the big picture, and knowing more accurately how to define one thing, helps define what is surround it, which make it easier to then find what surround that, and so on. Life isn't hiding from us, we are hiding from it, and when we decide come out of ourselves, we will find it.

If we feel stupid, it means that we figured out something so well that it seems glaringly obvious now. That should be looked at as a success, not a reason we should feel bad. Not only did we learn something, which is nice, we learned a lot, which is even better.

Whether if feels like it or not, we are always doing our current best, and our current best is always getting better. The reason we feel stupid, was because we can't believe we didn't know better, but that means, we didn't know better, and so shouldn't beat ourselves up over it. The fact that we all make mistakes anyway isn't an excuse for bad behavior. Knowing we shouldn't beating ourselves up for mistakes doesn't mean we don't have to fix problems we create, it means while we are fixing them, we shouldn't ruminate over wanting to go back in time or try to avoid them by hiding.

It seems, that it is not the present moment on its own that weights on us so heavily causing us trouble, but how we've tied that present moment to the future and past. We are more scared of what might happen if or when we get our mistakes thrown in our face later, than looking into the mistake itself and figuring out what went right and what went wrong.

Dr. Seuss said, "I have heard there are troubles of more than one kind. Some come from ahead and some come from behind. But I've bought a big bat. I'm all ready you see. Now my troubles are going to have troubles with me!"

What is this bat we can use to defend ourselves from shame that creeps up from the past, fear which haunts us from the future, and guilt which catches us in the now?

Dr. Seuss also said, "Sometimes the questions are complicated and the answers are simple."

Einstein and Dr. Seuss agree the hard part is figuring out the question, luckily there is more than one way to find it. Other people's experience seems just as well as mine to find good questions, the answers however, I think we all have to find on our own.

Dr. Seuss continues to answer the question, "The more that you read, the more things you will know. The more that you learn, the more places you'll go."

Albert Einstein said, "learning is experience. Everything else is just information." Information adds possibly real details to concepts in our mind, but learning is testing that information against life and finding out what parts of that information are real.

We all approach questions in different orders and in different ways, but if there is only one real answer, none of the imaginary ones will satisfy forever. As long as we don't settle for half-answers, we will all arrive at the same place, reality or objectivity.

My journey to figure out the mind and emotion, once I decided to make a serious study of it, started by searching neuroscience for the answer. That somehow lead me to philosophy, history, and then psychology. Because past experience greatly influences what we value, and I think the psychology class I took my first semester is college might be to blame for it being the last place I looked when I decided to search for the answer. The side of the big picture of life I had stumbled into the first eighteen years of my life, seem drastically different than the picture of life my psychology teacher portrayed. If I retook the exact same class now, I'm sure it would seem much different.

The order I searched out the question of mind and emotion ended up being helpful. Neuroscience narrowed the plausible possibilities of the wide range of philosophical thought. Philosophe gave me some context to the ideas psychological ideas wanted to solve, and why and when it separated from philosophe—what questions philosophe didn't seem to answer. History gave me some sense of which ideas in psychology would be most foundational, because they were themes that have come up in so many different forms throughout history in many different forms from myth, to meta-physics and etymology. Etymology was helpful to me to find what ideas words were created to describe, and how the meanings evolved to fit new discovered gaps in communication. Studying medicine allowed me to understand the divergence of psychology and psychiatry, and there I was full circle, back at neuroscience.

Which was the most helpful? Or which camp do I identify with? I have found great things in all of them, and comparing and contrasting the ideas they present, they have all inspired a lot of questions. Ironically though they were the question, most of all it was my own mind and emotion that helped me figure them out.

We all have insights or assumptions about some things we are more sure about than other things, and I hope when compared to the things you are most sure about in life, that what I propose in this book will fit right in. I have put the overview of the journey of connecting in a historical and philosophical basis, and now will introduce the details of the landscape and tools for this journey in the context of a brief history of psychology.

I would say the core question in psychology is, "What is driving me to do want what I want?"

Arthur Schopenhauer in 1839 said, "We can do what we wish, but we can only wish what we must." He postulated that our deepest drive or "will" was pointed towards survival.

A book published in 1901 from notes written by Fredrick Nietzsche was titled, <u>Will to Power</u>. "The higher man is distinguished from the lower by his fearlessness and his readiness to challenge misfortune." "I wish them the only thing that can prove today whether one is worth anything or not—that one endures." He postulated that our deepest drive or "will" was toward power.

In 1920 Sigmund Freud in "beyond the pleasure principle," added to his theory, that our deepest drives were Libido (sex-drive), and a competing instinct, the death drive.

In 1932 Otto Rank in his book <u>Art and Artist</u>, postulated that two drives governed us, psychological life, by which he meant individuation, and psychological death, by which he meant the sacrifice of individuation for collectivization.

In 1946 Viktor Frankl said in what was later published in Man's Search for Meaning, that our deepest drive was to find meaning. "In some ways suffering ceases to be suffering at the moment it finds a meaning, such as the meaning of a sacrifice." "Ever more people today have the means to live, but no meaning to live for."

I propose that are deepest drive comes from three separate parts of our mind, that in our intuition there is a drive towards seeing value and adding to it, and from our intellect there is a drive to apply logic and cut out the illogical. Lastly a will-power directed towards a balance of value and logic to produce contentment and composure. Like a gardener we are intuitively nurturing, and with our intellect carefully pruning, in a balance so that it can produce fruit and sustain us and bring us enjoyment.

The first two drives seem to oppose each other, one that adds and the other that subtracts, but that is only when either is used by itself. The third drive is what takes the best from the idea to add and idea to subtract and creates a balanced plan. In conversation, for it to be productive, we must allow all three drives to create a whole idea containing components to add, and components to subtract.

In facilitating connection with others through conversation, it is important to listen for the question they are asking, or trying to ask. We should be able to first identify what components they would like to add to a situation, and which they would like to subtract, and how they would like to go about doing that before adding in our thoughts. If they only propose a component or components to add or subtract, then we are likely to conflict because they are only engaging one of their three drives, and using only one of three functions. It would be more productive in the case of someone only presenting for example just a component to add, to ask what complimentary or associated components they would subtract, and then how would those work together into a plan. This might seem like an odd procedure, but it is important in order to figure out the context someone is speaking from by assessing the drives behind what they say. If someone is saying something very passionately but yet only appears to be engaging one drive in their thought, then there is a strong taboo that is preventing them from engaging all three drives that likely should be addressed first.

At times we listen to someone just enough to answer them, often we don't actually hearing every word someone says to us. It is easy to just listen until we feel we agree with them, and then just accept whatever they say. Or listen until we think we don't agree, and not accept anything from them. There is a marketing tactic to ask three questions you know someone will say yes to before asking them to buy something. It might be an effective way of selling people things they don't need, but that tactic doesn't have a place in actual connection. Love and connection are not gimmicky, they are real.

Chapter 10

If we ask someone a question, we should realize we are inviting them to nurture our idea, prune it, or both, and be willing to take it all. If someone else asks us a question, we should probably try to figure out if they want us to nurture, prune, or neither; even if there are things we want to nurture or prune, we have to be okay just listening. Taking criticism or even input can be hard, and some people might not be ready for it... we should be ready though.

Questions have the curious ability to keep us up at night, and as annoying as that is, it is probably because we feel committed to finding an answer in order to get something we want.

There seems to be an unspoken rule: to not burden others with extra questions about life to try to answer, especially if the other person can't see how the reward of answering it is worth it. The burden of a question about life is like slamming you finger in the door, it's a lot easier to accept when it just happened naturally, than to willingly put your hand out and close the door on it. Change is hard, and sometimes it's easier when something comes in and quickly forces us to change. Though a question about life might hurt like having the door slammed on your finger, in reality a door of opportunity is being opened. We all know we have to get over it when if we slam the door on ourself, but if someone else does it to us it's different, and so we should be careful.

With friends, sometimes we both stumble into the same question, and then have the opportunity to work together finding the answer. Once I have a conversation with a friend about a problem of mine, and after they say they have a similar one, it can more easily becomes a combined effort to find an answer. Once a question is already out in the open, new things I find about it are better received when I try to share them than the times when the topic was not a conversation beforehand. I notice when I am in the same situation I am more open to insight from the other person as well. The topic of giving constructive criticism doesn't seem to have a clear-cut answer, but that might be okay. I have found it more useful figuring out how to receive and use constructive criticism than to give it.

I try to be open with others about questions I have about the obstacles in my own life, particularly ones that I know involve me changing something about myself. I try to invite any insight anyone else have found about it, no matter how critical of me it might feel. With that attitude, when the criticism comes, no matter how constructive or not it feels, I try to take it well, thank them, and let them know if they think of anything else to let me know. This does two things, helps me gain insight, and creates an environment of learning where others feel more motivated to ask for constructive criticism too, because they see there is at least some reason to want criticism even if it is not very constructive.

Professional athletes, and really any professional that takes what they do seriously, pays money for the best people they can find to criticize them. When we seriously want to improve, we have a desire to know what to do to be better. We can either pay someone who knows the thing that we want to improve in really well, or we could find ten people to criticize us for free that are less qualified, and then spend the time to filter through what is constructive and what is not. There are many therapists who have their own therapist, because if we are smart, we know we don't have all the answers, and someone else might have some answers that we don't, ones that might make a big difference. It's hard to figure what you don't know you don't know. I try to surround myself with people I can trust their advice, but also I don't shy away from asking anyone and everyone else as well.

When I started racing motocross, my dad wasn't an expert motocross coach, but would watch other riders and tell me what differences he saw between me and those going faster than me. I started off always try to defend myself when he would tell me something I could change. To settle a dispute about a technique my dad and I disagreed on, we asked a pro rider to watch me and give me advice. All he said when I got done riding, was, "Just... go faster."

In a contemptuous way I went out, annoyed, and tried to prove to him that his advice was silly, and rolling my eyes and thinking sarcastically while back on the track, "Look, I'm 'just going faster!' Look, I'm going faster here, and here, and here!" I was so annoyed that I didn't realize, that I was suddenly going at least half again faster. That turned out to be some of the best advice I have ever received, and someone who has never ridden a bike or seen a motocross race could have told me the same thing.

I modified his advice a little to say, "Go at least a little bit faster through every turn, and down every straight." I started using landmarks on the track to note where I was letting of the gas and putting on the break, and just kept trying to hold on the gas just a tiny bit longer before braking in every corner. It became a game, and before I knew it, out of six classes of racing, I went from losing in the second lowest class, to doing pretty well in the second highest one. I know I could have continued the game of "just going faster" until I had made it to the top class, but I realized it wasn't worth the risk to my health, and probably wasn't the best career choice for me. I adapted the formula or game to other parts of my life, and found the same rewarding results.

There is no coach or consultant that give a hundred percent constructive or useful criticism, and there is no person that gives a hundred percent useless criticism. I have found it is sometimes hard to predict who will give the best advice for something, and so I just ask everyone and wait to be surprised. A lot of things in life feel a lot easier when we make them a game. Something I like to do is graph what advice I receive and how much I trust that person. The advice and level of trust usually have a correlation, and drawing a line from the people I trust the least to the most, it often points to something beyond the best advice I received. Sometimes the best advice we receive is good enough, but sometimes it's nice to see where the trend points to a new better answer might be.

There are many things we can do to prevent people criticizing us, but the things we do to block ourselves from criticism, also block us from constructive criticism. How else are we supposed to know what we don't know, unless we allow someone to tell us, even if they don't tell us in the best way?

I have found in everything someone says, there is at least some part of it to nurture, and something to prune, and that's okay. Even if is only gives us a small insight, its more than we had yesterday, and the more insight we have, the better we armed we are to find more.

Chapter 11

Our natural drives towards value and logic have seven different aspects of value they push towards. All seven are different but work together to maximize the value of each other. These aspects of value are also criteria for logic, and they could be used to assess anything. They are the following:

1) Functionality, 2) Accuracy, 3) Perspective, 4) Connection, 5) Stability, 6) Safety, 7) Excellence.

These drives are the means to an end, which is understanding of life, and ability to navigate in it, with the purpose of finding value and building on it. These drives work to find what is real, and what is valuable. Shame, guilt, and fear, are not real, and are not valuable.

Often it is easier to see what is holding us back than how to move forward. Moving forward happens naturally through trial and error, reflecting and remembering. After we take a step, then next step is almost implied. Though we cannot see the ultimate goal, the next step toward it isn't impossible to find.

What stops this natural process of progression, are shame, guilt, and fear.

Shame is the fear that something we had done, or was done to us, makes us unworthy of connection. Guilt is the fear that something we are doing, or is being done to us, makes us unworthy of connection. Anxiety is the fear that something we might do or might be done to us makes us unworthy or connection.

Shame, guilt and fear are all two edge swords, which will cut you just as well as others. In fact, when we constantly are swinging around that sword, since we are around ourselves more than around anyone else, we will probably get cut more than anyone else.

Shame, guilt and fear can seem motivating at times. I can look back on many things I have accomplished, and can see how proving I was worthy of connection was often at least a part of all of it. The problem however with shame as a motivation, is that the more we rely on it, the more real it becomes to us, and the more it becomes part of our life. The heart of shame is uncertainty and mistrust, which is the opposite of understanding. Shame is a personification of the pain of change. Yes, change produces momentary uncertainty, but then afterwards greater certainty. Shame on the other hand, although it can produce momentary comfort when we let it direct us, but it also then produces a greater and deeper-rooted uncertainty.

Running away from pain is different than running toward enjoyment. I don't think the impulse to shame, guilt, or cause fear in someone comes naturally, I think it is provoked. We pull out the double-edged sword of shame to defend ourselves from it.

What provokes us to pull out the sword and start cutting, is to defend our sense of self, self-esteem, sense of identity or sense of worth. Our sense of self is our imaginary friend that people keep walking over because they don't see it. We often think people see what they are doing when they walk on our sense of self, and then get triggered.

There are several fears that separate us from being able to connect with others. There are many possible fears, and unlike aspects of value or criteria for logic which are real, fear is not, and so they can only be loosely arranged into seven categories:

1)   The fear to be taken advantage of
2)   The fear to be deceived
3)   The fear to being uninteresting
4)   The fear to be unappreciated
5)   The fear of being controlled
6)   The fear to be abandoned
7)   The fear to be rejected

There always seems to be at least one reason to question our impulse to connect with others, or question someone else's impulse to connect with us. Letting fear paralyze us isn't going to help us do anything productive.

For example, a chicken is born with a fear of snakes, even the shape of them is enough to paralyze them with fear. You can take a chicken, lay it down, and draw a line in the dirt away from its beak, and it will lay there thinking it is a snake. I don't think we are as simple as chickens. I don't think we are born with fear of not being worthy of connection, but are blindsided by one of these fears, and then cautious guard against it until the fear is debunked.

"For once deceiv'd, was his; but twice were mine" is phrase from Iliad of Homer, written twenty-eight-hundred years ago and reiterated many times since. Heard now as, "Fool me once, shame on you, fool me twice, shame on me." For this reason, we avoid the shame repeating itself by being hypervigilant to it, in order to not be blindsided again. This creates a hypersensitivity to anything that could possibly turn into the same situation.

Maxims surface in our mind as tools to direct our investigation of things and situations, and some like Homer's, start us down the road of defending from shame instead of moving towards value and logic. One simple phrase can have a large impact on our life. Changing a mantra to, "just a little faster each lap," instead of, "vengeance is sweet," can make a big difference in the outcome of life. As good as short sweet phrases sound, we should be weary to assume we can sum up the great problems of life in one sentence...

To complicate matters of connection, apart from fears, we are plagued by taboos and ideals which restrict where we feel allowed to look for answers.

Similar to fears, taboos and ideals are not real, and so defining the categories is merely a sample idea of how common taboo groups might correspond to aspects of value and criteria of logic:

1)   To be ugly/broken
2)   To be stupid/oblivious
3)   To be uncommitted/lost
4)   To be needy/helpless
5)   To be mean/intrusive
6)   To be weird/paranoid
7)   To be fake/ridiculous

Categories of misguided ideals could be something like these:

1)   Be worth others paying attention to
2)   Be worth others trusting your insight
3)   Be worth others idealizing
4)   Be worth others responding to immediately
5)   Be capable of not having anything taken from them
6)   Be capable of being independent
7)   Be capable of fixing any problem

The problem of a taboo is that it tells us where we can and can't look for the solution to a problem, and makes contentment and composure seem like something we need other's permission to feel.

The feeling associated with things or situations can become either excitement or pain depending on whether an increase or decrease of shame, guilt or anxiety is felt. Also, the resistance to the taboo creates extra attention on it. In order to avoid using the tabooed tool or weapon, we have to make reasons why not to. Each time the tool the taboo was covering what seemed to be the right tool for the job and wasn't used because of the taboo, the assumptions substantiating why the taboo increases.

As soon as one of the many assumptions holding a taboo in place is debunked, likely the rest will unravel, and to make up for lost time, the tabooed thing will likely be over used. Its overuse will lead it to its eventual failure, because overuse implies use out of its context. Then all the reasons keeping it a taboo will likely come back. This process continues, back and forth we go, trying to figure out if it should be taboo or not, without first figuring out what it is, and what context it works in.

Chapter 12

There is a lot we find when we stop wanting things to be what they are not. Regardless of what we hope or want things to be, they are what they are, and when we stop wanting to find things different than they are, we will probably find them.

In our mind, not only do we conceptualize the world and other people, but we also conceptualize ourselves. Life is not actually contained in our mind as a concept—life is what it is. Shame drastically messes with our concept of life and of ourselves because shame makes us feel that all our self-worth is dependent on how we conceptualize ourselves and how others conceptualize us; because of this, our concepts of life and ourselves can become stronger than real life, and stronger than the real us.

It wasn't our idea that the concept of ourselves was so important. That was something we learned growing up as we heard others with such great passion many people emphasize "I, me, mine, and their name."

There is an important element of truth in the importance of "I," because we are the only thing we have control over, but at a young age we likely learned that "I" was important so that we could become worthy of love and connection.

The concept of "I" was not the only concept that was terribly incomplete—we make a concept of everything in life, and those concepts all start just as crude and misleading as our concept of ourself. Because experience is misleading, we shouldn't hold onto our crude concepts of life and ourselves—we should let them change and be refined.

It would be hard not to notice that "I love you," is often followed by, "...because (something to do with their concept of us in their mind)." We can appreciate someone for doing something dependable, sincere, thoughtful, or whatever, and those can be reasons why we trust someone, but it shouldn't be a condition for loving them.

If we made a list of the reasons we think people love us, and then ask someone who loves us if they still would if we stopped being those things. I can only speak for myself, but if someone I love suddenly stopped being dependable, sincere, thoughtful, or whatever, I would want to give them more love, because I would assume they need it, and I would try to figure out what was going on, so I could try to help. I have often felt a lot of love in my lowest times, when I felt I didn't have much to give. If connection is synergy, then it makes sense that it seems sometimes harder to figure out where we can add our energy to someone else's when they seem to be doing it efficiently themselves.

If your experience is like mine, we have been learning love backwards, we feel we have to hide our imperfections in order to be worthy of connection, when really the imperfections are where we need the synergy of connection most, and where it most easily can come.

We have to be willing to challenge what we think we know, or we may never really know.

In an Essay on Criticism, by Alexander Pope, he says, "A little learning is a dangerous thing."

Why is that?

For example, if all you knew about aspirin, was that it could damage the stomach, you would have no reason to think that giving it to someone having a heart attack would help, because all you know is the smaller reason not to. The damage to the stomach is true, but not as important piece of the picture as how it can break up a clot in the heart. The damage to the stomach is very small in comparison, and can be countered by taking it with food. We don't know what we don't know. We also don't know what we think we know that we are really wrong about.

Singing the American national anthem as a child, I apparently didn't hear the words "dawn's early," what I heard was, "dawnserly." I thought for a very long time that "dawnserly" was an adverb to describe the magic of knowing the sun was rising, but where the evidence of it was imperceptible, because it happened so slowly and quietly. It made a lot of sense in thinking of the American revolution as slowly and quietly being born in the hearts of brave Americans willing to die for what they felt was right... It wasn't until I used "dawnserly" in a sentence and someone asked what I just said, that I found out it wasn't a word.

Because of that experience and others, now, in my database of knowledge, I try to label each assumption with how confident I am in it. If all things we think we know are used with the same confidence and enthusiasm despite how much knowledge we actually have about them, then what we know little about, will get us in more trouble than what we know well. For example, as a six or seven-year-old child I knew a little about wind resistance, just enough to feel confident it was a good idea to jump off the roof of my house with an umbrella...

If all we know about shame, is that it can be used to get people to do what we want, because it seems to motivate us. Or, if all we know about shame is that we don't want to feel it, and distraction helps not feel it. Either of these little bits of knowledge are fairly dangerous things.

But how else do we gain knowledge other than little bits at a time?

We are all pioneering our way forward through trial and error. There is a formula however to get the best results:

1) Identifying all the possible things that could be added to the situation to make it better.
2) Identifying all the things that could be taken away from the situation to make it better
3) Crossing out all the things you want others to do, and then from the things you want to do, take the top five or ten percent of the things to possibly add and subtract, and then figure out a way to work them together into a plan.

What comes out of this formula should be tested to confirm it has actually improved the situation. We can run the formula as many times as we want.

It is very straining on the mind to feel it has to accept and keep a hundred percent of the random thoughts that arise, especially since one part of our mind thinks the complete solution is to add, and the other part thinks it is to subtract.

What to do with what other people say can be an obstacle, if we feel we have to accept or reject a hundred percent of what other people say. We can run what others say through the same formula, look for what they want to add, what they want to subtract, and take the top five or ten percent of each.

Before we learned about shame, naturally we held on to the what seemed useful, and discarded what didn't seem useful. Now, the fear of shame scares us into holding tightest to the least helpful, least true thing in life which is shame. A phrase that has likely evolved from Sun Tzu's Art of War, written in 6th century BC, Puzo and Coppola wrote in a 1974 movie: "Keep your friends close but your enemies closer."

Likely we have come to believe that our mind and emotions are at war. Somehow, we have embraced the idea that our most destructive thoughts and emotions should be kept closest, so we can monitor and manage them more carefully. It seems we are either trying to hold shame tightly as a prisoner of war... which kills us from the inside. Or run to meet shame in battle... killing us from the outside. What would happen if we just didn't try to capture or chase shame?

A sense of self is an imaginary friend, and shame is an imaginary enemy, and there is no limit to what imaginary enemies can do to attack. We often forget that our happiest times are when we are caught up in the moment and not thinking about ourselves.

Marcus Aurelius a 1st century king and philosopher said in his book Meditations, "If you are distressed by anything external, the pain is not due to the thing itself, but to your estimate of it; and this you have the power to revoke at any moment."

What if someone came up and handed you twenty dollars, how would you feel?

Now imagine that you find out, that on a dare, the person that gave you the twenty dollars was asked to find the stupidest person they could, and give them twenty dollars. How would you feel then?

That free twenty dollars couldn't hurt your wallet, but depending on the context, could hurt your sense of self. What Marcus Aurelius said, is that the tendency to estimate the worth of things in comparison to our own worth, brings pain; because when compared to our worth, we will feel the thing is not worth us, or that we are not worth it. Rarely would we feel our worth and the other thing or person's worth are the same, and so anxiety about possibly finding out we are nothing worth the thing or person is scary.

Self-esteem is just the temporary absence, repression or distraction from the feeling of shame. The only thing real about shame is our reaction to it, which is within our control. Not much needs to be understood about it other than we shouldn't react to things that aren't real.

Shame, guilt, and fear are learned ideas. They are ideas forced on us in the form of ideals and taboos, which are claims of value or logic that cannot be tested.

For example, various people have told me not to wear white after Labor Day. Also, various people have told me not to put tin foil in the microwave... Of course, I put both to the test. Wearing white was fine, but the tin foil caught fire and possibly did permanent damage to the microwave...

Turns out not wearing white after Labor Day is likely just a silly taboo, and the warning of putting tin foil in the microwave has actual value and logic behind it.

If I say, you should feel bad or be ashamed because... (insert whatever irrational and untestable claim), what do you do with that?

Something that has actual value, it's value is augmented when logic is applied to it. Since value is assessed by intuition and felt as emotion, the way to know whether it is a real emotion instead of a fleeting feeling is to apply logic to it—if the logic destroys it, it was just a fleeting feeling. Shame is felt as a feeling, but it can be shown to be as hollow and unreal as it is when logic is applied and it falls flat.

Not all feelings are real communication from our intuition, some are just triggers in our ego, or identity.

Chapter 13

Our mind has the ability to find value and apply logic. Other people can offer us good questions to ask and give help in directions to look for answers, but learning really happens when we apply what we feel and think is the answer, and then afterward reflecting on where our understanding worked and where it was lacking. We shouldn't let something or someone bypass our own ability to look and feel for ourselves, because there's no way to skip the testing part of the learning phase.

If something has objective value or logic, it should independently be assessable to see by everyone eventually. What is real doesn't need to be defended. I believe the law of gravity is real, not because Isaac Newton had convincing arguments for it, but because I tested it. I'm sure anyone else who wants to test gravity will come up with a similar conclusion, that there is a force pulling things down.

Heraclitus, a fifth century BC philosopher said, "Though wisdom is common, yet the many live as if they had a wisdom of their own." Gravity doesn't do one thing for a certain person and a different thing for someone else, and neither doesn't anything else real in life.

There is an ancient parable about several blind men feeling an elephant, all think it is something different. One grabs the tail and thinks it is a snake, another grabs a leg and thinks it's a tree. The reality whether or not any could perceive it, was that it was an elephant. Once we cross at least the first three bridges over the pitfalls to connection, we would see the whole elephant, even if someone was holding the tail swore it was a snake. After crossing all four bridges we would not only know what it was, but also not be angry or laugh when someone calls it a snake. To add to that, we might be able to calmly and sincerely ask a question to help them figure out what it is on their own.

"Oh wow, you found a snake, could you bring it here and show me?"

"I can't... it seems to be attached to something..."

"Attached to what?"

After following the tail to where it connects, "Attached to a wall..."

"If that's the case, it might actually be an elephant, to check if that is true, you could follow the wall down and see if it starts to feel like a tree trunk."

"Oh wow, it does, you were right! I think it's an elephant."

If someone really wants to know, they will feel out the whole elephant—it's not like people can't figure things out without our help. We can help, but being pushy isn't helping.

For example, my claim that tin foil and a microwave don't go together should be tested if that information is important to you. Similarly, my theory of a map of mind and emotion should be tested. Just as in the microwave the tinfoil will show sparks after a few seconds, insights should spark in your mind as what I propose resonates with what your experience has been.

Not testing the assumption about tin foil and microwaves likely won't have as big an effect as not testing the false assumption that we shouldn't actually feel bad when we fail, or that we don't have to be perfect to be loved. A lot of our emotional life often is built on assumptions that are dangerous and untested.

Realizing that everything we think is just assumptions of what actually is, and often those assumptions were not ones we made from trial and error, but from what others have told or think we saw other people do. This is why finding what is real is completely up to us, because we must take our own assumptions and test them, then make better ones and test them.

Shel Silverstein in a poem entitled, "The Voice" said,

"There is a voice inside of you
That whispers all day long
'I feel this is right for me
I know that this is wrong.'
No teacher, preacher, parent, friend
or wise man can decide
what's right for you—just listen to
The voice that speaks inside."

That voice inside of us that has the power to be the final say in what we do is us; that's who we are, so we should probably listen to it. Yes, the artist function inside of us has a voice, and the engineer function as well, but it is the executive that has the final say.

Like the poem says, we might only feel what is good, and have a vague idea what is wrong, but we are figuring it out one day at a time, and that's okay; life is meant to be lived one day at a time anyway.

I don't think life needs any instructions to figure it out—it's kind of just a guess and check sort of game. The process of guess and check is a lot different than the process try and fail, because when we guess and then check, we get excited to guess again. When we try and fail, failing doesn't motivate us to keep trying.

In life there are many instances of unexpected learning, where we thought we were learning one thing, and after testing it, we found out we were learning something else. It's impossible to know exactly what we want to learn and how to figure it out, until we know it... but then the process is over. So, unexpected learning is the only way we ever learn, and that's okay.

Karen Horney, a psychanalyst said "Fortunately psychoanalysis is not the only way to resolve inner conflicts. Life itself still remains a very effective therapist... The therapy effected by life itself is not, however, within one's control."

Life is real, but the concept of life in our mind is mingled with things that are not real, like fears, ideals and taboos.

Once the idea of shame is introduced, and while entertained as being real, it grows. At times others shame us, other times we shame ourselves, this means it is possible for shame to always be present, which can lead us to feeling like we are drowning in it... all the time. Similar to a person drowning, we clutch and flail, and in the panic, find ourselves pushing someone else down to try to get our head above the water... the imaginary water of self-esteem.

One wholly accepted ideal or taboo held on without end, is enough to unravel our sanity.

Brené Brown in her book: The Gifts of Imperfection, speaking of one specific ideal, perfectionism said, "Perfectionism is a self-destructive and addictive belief system that fuels this primary thought: If I look perfect, and do everything perfectly, I can avoid or minimize the painful feelings of shame, judgment, and blame."

At first an ideal might seem appealing, who would not want to do everything to perfection, and thereby not have anything that can be criticized? But an ideal is a target not a measuring stick. Of course we will never be an ideal, but it would be silly not to shot for it.

We could only even come close to an ideal if that were the only thing we put our energy into. Doing our best is one thing, but doing our best at only one thing at the cost of all others is different; this is what we do when we feel that there is only one ideal people are looking for.

"I throw perfect parties," "I deliver perfect jokes," "I am always supportive," are all identities, they are all different hats we put on when that hat is appropriate, but there is no "one hat to rule them all." We can match the hat for the weather, but it's impossible to match the weather for the hat... but that doesn't stop us from trying sometimes.

The false idea that holding one ideal well enough is all that matters is not easily debunked—all we have to do it open a magazine to see an ideal model that receives money and fame without saying or doing anything except just standing there. Not to mention how much seems to be possible with the ideal bank account. Though we know focusing on chasing just one ideal is not the long-term answer, doing it as short-term fix is very appealing.

Connection is not a mere feeling. There are times when we pretend to listen to someone but aren't. There are times when we are trying not to listen, but then end up hearing what they say and thinking about it positively later. We can feel we are connecting when we are not, and actually be connecting when we don't feel it. Trying to find a way to confirm we are being seen, heard or understood leads us to treating the connection as the goal and the person as a means to get there. Connection is the means and being able to really be present with others is the goal.

Connection is a subtle synergy, it is also intuitive and automatic. It is more apparent when it is severed than when it is created. Just like a friendship, we may remember the moment we realized we were friends, but not the moment when the friendship started.

Since a by-product of connection is a feeling of self-worth, it is tempting to gauge our connection with someone else by how we feel about ourselves. Connection is not felt as much as disconnection is, which is the feeling we often associate with shame. We have to get passed the tendency to try to measure connection by the absence of shame so that we make the person the focus, not our shame.

If shame were actually real, it would be logical to just let shame train us to be ideal, because then we wouldn't have to worry about it. Well, shame isn't real, and so listening to it won't work. Shame tells us being human is shameful, the way we dress, the way we walk, talk, and chew our food, even the way we feel and perceive is shameful.

"One man runs to his neighbor because he is looking for himself, and another because he wants to lose himself. Your bad love of yourselves makes solitude a prison for you." -Friedrich Nietzsche

In the course of life as we stumble across the same things as others, we naturally have things to talk about. True connection is spontaneous. We have the whole world in common, there shouldn't need to be any pretense to connect. We would see the world better if we weren't walled off from it by shame.

Reaching an ideal is not the way to connect, and avoiding a taboo is not either. For example, being needy is a taboo, which could make us not want to initiate conversation in order to not seem needy... Not offending people is an ideal, but thinking that initiating a conversation could seem like we are implying that they are not confident enough to do it themselves...

It might seem crazy, but if we actually wrote down what our shame tells us, it would show how ridiculous, counterproductive, and wrong it is.

Once we let go of the idea that reaching ideals and avoiding taboos is the answer, that wall of shame, guilt and anxiety between us and everything else disappears, and as naturally and imperceptibly as dew collects from the cool morning air, we will find each other.

Chapter 14

Mankind has figured out how to place satellites in space, moving at eighteen-thousand miles an hour, in perfect balance with the gravity of the earth and the speed it's rotating. To add to that great feat, while up there hurling through space, it processes data sent to it, making four billion calculations a second. So, why we can't we seem to figure out why being vulnerable with people we claim to trust is so difficult?

People have broken through the barriers which separate us from outer space, yet there are barriers between our heart and mind still keep us locked in our own little world.

In 1789 a classification of chemical elements, "the Periodic table," began to be put together. Understanding the basic building blocks the more complicated molecules of life are built on, has increased the ability of chemists, biologists and engineers to understand the world around us, and innovate and explore new things. In that same venue, I propose a similar classification of the components of the mind and emotion—the building blocks both the tools and weapons of connection and conflict arise from.

The periodic table is arranged in columns where each element in a row has the same electrical charge, giving us a really good idea of how different elements will interact when mixed. The right most column is the noble gases, which have no electric charge. Elements combine to have balance, with a "noble number or ratio of electrons to protons."

This portion of the book is meant to be an in-depth study, focused on a proposed blue print of the mind and emotions, composed of components of perception and decision. This map of the anatomy of the psyche should resonate with your past and present experience in context of emotions, and the process of thought.

I am not suggesting what types of people will interact well together, nor am I suggesting what types of things a person should do. My endeavor is to frame or categorize the fundamental aspects which value has, and how that matches up with the anatomy of our psyche.

This book is not an idea of mental health habits, a modality of therapy, or a suggestion of a social contract, but rather a fundamental theory containing the tools or building blocks by which all matters of the mind could be approached.

This will be principally focused on aspects of value, and criteria of logic, and how they combine to make intrapersonal and interpersonal tools. Furthermore, this will be a map of what

I propose to be the anatomy of mind and emotion, which will define the relationship between emotions, intellect, intuition and will-power.

Despite how uncontrolled or odd our thoughts and emotions can feel at times, our mind is our own, and we are allowed to open it up and see what's inside. What we find when we do, is that our intellect is not a prison, our intuition is not a mystery box of crazy ideas, and our emotions are not a rollercoaster ride we never signed up for—they are the tools we have to understand and operate in life.

Socrates said, "the unexamined life is not worth living." I would modify his statement a little to say, "the unexamined life is not living."

It is surprising how much of our daily life can be carried out without thinking about it, as if were running on auto-pilot. The word "conscious" means "to know," and it seems there is quite a bit in our life that is carried along unconsciously. How much of our life is examined or conscious?

C.G. Jung said, "until you make the unconscious conscious, it will control your life, and you will call it fate."

Fate is everything outside of our control that happens, choice is what we do with what we have control over. It is not readily apparent what we have control over and what we do not, but looking into our actions, can help us separate them.

What we value, shapes how we see things, and how we see things, shapes what we choose to do. What we do in turn, shapes what we see, and what we see, determines what value we find.

What we value is not always the same as other people on the surface level, it can even seem that what we value and what someone else values are opposites sometimes. When we go deeper, there seem to be a set number of fundamental aspects of value that all adjectives we use to describe things fit into. For example, gold. It is brilliant, malleable, doesn't rust, isn't toxic, and is rare, which has given it value across cultures and throughout time.

Diamonds and gold are quite different, opposite even in some respects, where one is malleable, the other is one of the hardest substances on earth, but both overlap in brilliancy, not rusting, not being toxic and being rare. The question: "Which is better, diamonds or gold?" would have to be qualified by defining which aspect of value was being compared. Someone could say that gold has no aesthetic value for them which is up to them, but its value as being malleable is a fact. One gram of gold can be flattened into a sheet one square meter wide, which is much better than most everything else in the world. Anyone could compare and contrast gold against other metals for malleability and come to the same conclusion.

It seems anything can be labeled with a money value, or attention factor. Going deeper than aspects such as monetary value, popularity or entertainment value, we find what influences someone to pay what they do for something, or why it gets the popularity it does. Previous experience will greatly shape what we value until we go deep below the subjective surface-level value we see, all the way down to the bedrock or foundational aspects of value which are objective or real.

I propose all instances of value we see fall under one of seven different categories:

1) Functionality/Purpose
2) Accuracy/Reproducibility
3) Exploration/Adventure/Perspective/Context
4) Connection/response/continuity
5) Stability/Strength/Resolve
6) Protection/Preservation/Security
7) Excellence/Ability to overcome/catalyst

Each aspect of value can only be assessed individually. We cannot determine at the same time whether something is accurate or stable and also adventurous. Adventure means going into uncharted territory, and so there would be no way of knowing whether it was going to be stable, or way of knowing whether you can accurately say what you will find on the adventure. However, something with value as a whole, will have value in each of the seven aspects. In order to compare and contrast whether to do something or not, we could use all seven aspects of value to determine the overall utility of a decision.

Even though we know we should take time and really think things through, instead of assess one by one the seven different aspects of value we see, often there is so much going on with the pressures of life, that we feel we only have time to assess one or maybe two aspects of value for a decision. Even if we do have the time, we usually fixate on just one aspect of things, and get distracted from the rest.

In an argument, likely each person only sees one or two aspects of value in the situation, and since they don't agree, they are probably different aspects.

An example of one aspect of value influencing a decision. Some people build a house out of material that is easiest to work with, so that the job can go faster. Some people build a house out of the strongest material, so that it will last the longest. Some build a house out of the cheapest material. Some people build a house out of the rarest material in order to... I don't know, be adventurous maybe. And some people try to build a house out of the best combination of strength, ease and affordability.

It is nice to have a house that is unique, because it could possibly spur conversation, or create a sense of separation from other parts of our life so that we feel at home while at home. Uniqueness is an aspect to factor in, but probably not at the expense of other aspects of value. If we looked at just uniqueness for building a house, one of the most unique things anyone could build their house out of would be Lithium, or solid metal sodium, but if you did that, as soon as it rained, not only would your house be gone, but because of the explosive reaction with water, you would be gone as well. Uniqueness in the case of building a house plays a part, but is not the most pivotal aspect of value.

What prevents us from seeing the most pivotal aspect of value at play in a situation is probably our past experience. What we value shapes how we see things, and how we see things shapes what we choose to do. What we do, in turn shapes what we see, and what we see determines what value we find. This can create quite a bias in our perception of things.

For example, if you just experienced a situation where you regret not holding your ground, and now someone is trying to sway your opinion. With that as the context of experience, accepting the other person's idea, would feel like you are not holding your ground, and in danger of losing control of the situation again.

If you felt your self-worth was less because you weren't strong when you needed to, then anything remotely close to the same situation could feel like another incidence of not being strong enough.

Now, imagine that the person trying to sway your opinion, just had an experience where they felt that no one cared about they think. And maybe they felt since it was their idea, the rejection was of them and their idea. They likely in that case regret not presenting their idea clearly or persuasively enough. This would mean it would be very probable that they feel their self-worth is dependence on validation of their ideas from others, and will be sensitive to us not wanting to listen or accept their idea.

In this case, both are perceiving a radically different events; one leaves feeling harassed and the other leaves feeling rejected, when in reality both naively entered the situation with a very biased perception. We can't always second guess our perception of everything in life, but if at the onset of a conflict we were to start resolving it by challenging our assumptions, we would both resolve conflicts quickly and learn consistently.

We seem to always be carrying the last major conflict in our lives, and looking at all the sequent situations as a way to solve it. Until that major conflict is solved, our interactions with people are greatly influenced by the question our last conflict proposed. We often try in our current situation what we think could have been the solution to our last major conflict, despite how applicable it may be in our current situation.

For example, even at our best thinking, when we know there is a balance between discretion and openness, if our last conflict seemed to be caused by not expressing ourself, we then compensate and are too open. If in our last conflict someone threw something in our face we wish we hadn't told them, we will likely overcompensate and just not say anything. Both mitigations due to past experiences are not necessarily fair to the person in our current situation.

There is a saying, "To someone with a hammer in their hand, everything starts to look like a nail." A hammer is a good tool, but shouldn't be our only tool. We should have our tool bag complete with all the tools of life, and figure out what tool is best for what we want to do. Otherwise we will just pass from phase to phase—the diet phase, the overworking phase, the clinging phase, and any other compensation other than the right tool for the right job.

How do we determine what tool we approach a situation with?

We typically solve problems with what we have seen work for others, what has worked for us before, or most likely just the tool we are best at using. History has shown that the country with the one tool that beats all the rest, can take over a considerable portion of the world. The long sword, long bow, short sword, bronze sword, chariot, and faster horses, ship or tanks, each in their time were the one tool to rule them all. Each aspect of value is a way to find an answer or solution.

In a situation it could be that we will figure out exactly what is going on by dissecting it into its components. It could be that connecting with the right person will provide the answer. It could be just continuing pushing forward. Etc. If we are really good at even just one of those, that usually seems to solve a lot of problems, which means there is little incentive to develop more ways to approach a situation.

In our lives, we learn how to use new tools out of necessity when a conflict arises, or through play in a simulated conflict like a game, sport or pretend.

Competition in all its forms seems to be a game of one or multiple of seven aspects: utilization, accuracy, wit, reaction-time, endurance, efficiency, or problem solving.

Using basketball as an example, the key to winning might be:

1) Utilization of picks and post-ups.
2) Making a higher percentage of the shots taken.
3) Being aware of who is where on the court, and what plays the other team will use.
4) Quick passes and making yourself open to be passed to.
5) Endurance; just outrunning the other team.
6) Quickly getting on the ball for rebounds and boxing out.
7) Reading the players on the other team, and considering the obstacles. Looking at strengths of your team to figure out how to overcome what they will try to use to stop you.

With seven quite different aspects to the sport of basketball, which do you make the focus of the limited time available to practice?

In a relationship, maybe one person is gauging the interest of the other by how constant the contact is, meanwhile the other person maybe being looking at the quality of each interaction. This would mean one person is texting all day, and the other doesn't always have something really meaningful to reply, and might get stressed out trying to keep up. Meanwhile, the other person will ruminate why there is a lag in response.

In a team at work, maybe you want to increase the efficiency of what resources are already being used, and someone else wants to explore other possible resources.

Where we search first for the solution to a question can lead us in different directions, but should ultimately lead to the same conclusion, if there actually is an objective answer. If there is not an objective or actual answer, then there would be no point in preferring your approach over someone else's.

Though our search for the answer might lead us in a different direction than someone else at first, and even if it seems to conflict, once each aspect is assessed, and each criteria of logic applied, you will be able to see where they got their answer, and be closer to finding an objective conclusion.

When working with others, the best aspect to focus on first, might likely just be whichever everyone can agree on. When tackling a project ourselves, we can look at it from all seven of those aspects and figure out which one is most pivotal to do first.

Chapter 15

There is a book where the main character has to pass through every possible trial, just to get rid of something dangerous he didn't invent or even want. We find ourselves in a similar situation, except minus the elves, wizards or volcano to throw the source of the problem into.

We didn't invent the ambiguous and volatile sense of self-worth. We also didn't invent how our sense of self-worth seems relative to someone else's, or dependent on what someone else says or even implies. Worse, we didn't invent the idea that some people are worth connecting with and others not.

"In the social jungle of human existence, there is no feeling of being alive without a sense of identity." -Erik Erikson

The problem the idea of self-worth creates is only apparent when it's not in our favor. But is a relative self-worth in anyone's favor? I believe it's possible we can evolve past making life a social jungle of mere fleeting sensations and hysteria.

The idea of self-worth or self-esteem keeps us in competition with all the people we want to connect with, where when we win, we are worth connecting to and they are not, and when they win, we aren't worth connecting with but they are.

Just as the main character in that popular fiction story finds out quite early in the adventure, the dangerous ring he has been given also has a power which makes some situations quite a bit more convenient, so to self-esteem which is dangerous seems to make some situations easier. Whereas the ring enabled the main character to be invisible, our sense of self-worth makes us feel seen, heard and valued.

We find the idea of relative self-worth to be convenient sometimes. We want to be seen… if we are seen doing something that will prove our self-worth, so that we will feel worth connecting to. Otherwise, if we are doing something that proves our shame, we want to be invisible. This dichotomy complicates things, because what we do is a result of us seeing value in it which not everyone will also see the same value, and since nothing we do is perfect anyway, everything we do is liable to cause us shame. This means we switch back and forth fairly frequently whether we want to hide or be seen.

At times, we think we have what it takes to prove our self-worth, which would mean we are allowed to connect… but ends up being at the expense of inadvertently proving everyone else isn't worth connecting to, or that they are lucky to be able to connect with someone more capable or selfless than them.

It's not intentional of course, but comes out unless much care is taken to avoid it.

What we are usually trying to prove is that we are selfless, capable, or both. Trying to prove that you are selfless is ironic, because a selfless person doesn't do nice things in order to be seen, they do it just because it seems good to do. Proving capability is equally as ironic, because for someone to say you are capable, it would mean they would have to admit they were less capable than you.

It is unlikely someone would want to sacrifice part of their sense of self to give you more. Just as many sports fans leave a game where their team lost, still saying their team is better. We can't control what someone thinks, and there seems to be no benefit in doing it either.

I think we are more likely to enjoy what we are doing, if we focus on figuring out what we actually want to do, instead of what we think we should prove. Rarely is it immediately apparent in a situation what we want to do before considering what the situation actually is, and what can or should be done. By reframing the situation in reference to all seven aspects of value, we will know better what the best options are, and which we actually see value in.

Sometimes it seems that what we authentically want to do, either doesn't seem to prove our self-worth to others, or even diminishes it. I remember feeling in high school frustrated that it seemed every girl wanted to wear a football jersey, it didn't even seem to matter who the owner of the jersey was or if they even got game-time. Early in high school I was already racing motocross at a college level, and couldn't imagine any girl wanting to wear my racing jersey at school on race day.

There is often pressure to prove what others seem to think is worth proving, and it leads us to doing and saying things we don't actually see value in. It is not a genuine pursuit of value which leads a child to steal, vandalize or hurt, it is social pressure pushing on their sense of self-worth.

If we put so much effort into proving things we don't really see value in, just so we can be worth connecting to, will that change once we connect? Or why are we willing to do things we don't see value or logic in, if the synergy of connection will just amplify what we are doing that we already didn't see value in?

Understanding of the purpose and conditions of connection is not a prerequisite for connection. The journey to find understanding of the purpose and conditions of connection can help us find and challenge the assumptions that have got in the way of our innate ability to connect.

What is connection?

In short, I would say connection is synergy—where two hearts or minds is better than one in a situation. Not just better in immediately apparent results, but in all seven aspects of value. Connection doesn't have to be in person or even in the moment—just knowing someone will be excited to hear what we are doing, motivates us and even inspires more ideas because we consider what they would say if they were there in the moment.

Sometimes although doing something yourself may seem immediately more functional, slowing down and helping someone else be involved will help them and likely you as well later. Sometimes

What makes connection?

Connection seems to be a shared experience, seeing the same instance of value, both people applying logic to it, and both investing will-power into it.

Something that adds to connection, is that the same instance of value can be seen a little different, and those differences in perspective can be shared leading to increased understanding and ability to add to it.

In finance the word appreciate means to raise in value, or to build on a principal balance. Two people investing in the same asset of life, increases its potential to grow.

How do we see what instance of value someone else is seeing?

We see things kind of like a camera. A camera combines three different layers of film, each having reacted to a specific color range of light, red, green and blue, which combined gives us a picture in all its detail and colors.

Unlike the camera, we can only use one layer of film at a time. Apart from three different color film layers, a camera has several different lenses to use, anything from wide angle or macro, to telescopic. Apart from taking a picture from the same angle as someone else, in order to see the same thing as someone else, we must use the same colored layer of film, and the same lens.

I propose there are seven different emotional lenses, each specialized for seeing different aspects of value. Also, that there are three systems of the psyche, or layers of film, each able to perceive different colors of life. It is our task to use all seven lenses and all three layers of film, and try to see things from as many angles as possible, to understand the whole big picture of life.

We can survive with one lens and one layer of film, but when we have the capacity to prosper or thrive in life, what meaning would it have to settle for merely surviving?

The fewer lenses and layers of film we use, the smaller portion of life we will see, and the less likely it is, that what we see will match up with anyone else.

Each emotional lens and each systems of the psyche combine to make a tool. When used outside its proper application or zone of utility, that tool becomes a weapon. The general categories of tools which line up with the systems of the psyche are learning, supporting, and appreciating.

The generalized weapons which come from the different systems of the psyche are:

Shame, which is vindictive.
Guilt, which is commandeering.
Fear, which is hostile.

We are born fearless, shameless, and guiltless, and maybe that is why we don't know what to do sometimes, because we weren't born knowing how to deal them and they come up so often now.

Instead of moving towards value and logic, at times we find ourselves running away from the fear of losing connection with others. Running away from where we think we want to be least is different than running towards where we want to be most.

What do we really want in life? Is it the same as what everyone else wants?

Looking into the context of excitement shows a common trend.

Excitement tends to result in a combination of three things:
1) a reward we want,
2) a plan to get it that seems possible
3) a response to indicate progress towards it.

When those three criteria are met, the time, energy, emotion and thinking used, don't seem to bother us, and we generally feel excited. Whereas, even if we can see a favorable reward, if we don't feel capable of attaining it, or there seems to be no way of knowing if we are progressing toward it, any energy spent on it seems exhausting, and a general feeling of boredom or frustration likely sets in.

Sharing excitement seems to be instinctual. "Mom! Dad! Look what I made!" As children, the reward often we were looking for from the art project or whatever we had done, was recognition or validation. I think, though we try to add a lot of complexity to our instinct to share excitement, at its root, not much has changed since we were young.

Making interpersonal connection, we can use the same formula as excitement: 1) synergy of feeling, 2) synergy of ideas, or 3) synergy of action.

What types of reward are we looking for? Money? Power? Fame? Those are typical things people seem to want, but couldn't that merely just be adding one more step to what we really want, recognition and validation?

Maybe the question is, "in order to form a connection, what does the other person want recognized or validated?"

The specific positive adjectives someone often uses in conversation are probably a good indication of what someone would want validated, or the opposite of the negative adjectives someone complains about.

Sometimes we want validation and recognition so much, that although telling someone what they want to hear is not actually validation, it is merely endorsement, but since it feels similar enough, in desperation we are sometimes content with either...

I think the reason we want validation is because we are exploring life, and just want confirmation that what we are finding really exists. We get a sense early on in life that it is possible to do things wrong, usually because others point it out, making us feel broken. "What were you thinking?!" "That's not what that is used for!" "You're an idiot!"

Because of so much extra uncertainty being forced on us, the easiest way to not feel broken would be do what others say, so that they don't point things out. At some point after trying to just do what people say to avoid feeling broken, we realize people seem to never run out of things to tell us to do, and some of those things we don't actually want to do. It shouldn't be so hard to just make people happy, but it is; we should cut ourselves a lot more slack for the heroic efforts we have already made to make people happy, it has just been slightly misdirected because it was under the assumption that value is subjective, but now knowing the best way to make other people happy is to no second-guess ourselves, and do what we see has logic and value.

There is a mantra we are born with, "my best will always be enough, I will always be enough," and when that mantra fails us, life stops making sense. Any meaning we try to find in life without that core maxim just gets dark and confusing.

Statements like, "I don't even know you anymore," "You're a disappointment, I just can't believe you would do that," are too big of ideas for a young mind to handle. These statements and many more go against our inner mantras that love is always enough, and that we are always enough. Each situation seems to prove our inner mantra right or wrong. Having our core assumption so often challenged makes life very uncertain, and allows that uncertainty to go all the way to our core.

In the process of life, we are learning and finding instances of value and adding to it, and what we want is validation that the process of life is working. Our core assumptions of meaning and purpose in life can't be built upon until they are solid enough, because if our core assumptions are wrong or shaky, then all the assumptions built on top of them would be wrong or shaky also. It is very scary to think that all the assumptions we are making could completely change upon finding out our core assumptions are wrong, this is why we want others to tell us that what we think is at least close enough.

Whether we realize it or not, we are in fact always learning and adding value, because we are always gathering data through our experiences, despite whether that data was pursued or forced on us by life. Even if that data is skewed by bias, it's only a matter of time before the trend of our bias becomes very apparent and we improve it. The fact that we are in a process of learning and growing that only moves forward isn't readily apparent, because our results in life seem to go up and down. This is for several reasons, but the greatest is the fact that the more aware we become of our situation, since pain is the easiest to see, and doesn't involve gratitude or long-term thinking, we will likely become more aware first of the pain we hadn't noticed before.

Because we often don't realize that we are always doing better than we were yesterday, we get embarrassed when we think instead of learning or adding value, we are getting learning lies and losing value, which is the root of shame, guilt and anxiety.

Fear of being stupid or heartless seem to be the main fears. However, being stupid is not actually possible, because once you realize that what you thought is actually not correct, you now are smarter than you were. In fact, the less you can believe how you would do something so stupid, means that now, what you were oblivious to, you are now very aware. You would have to be smart to have a valid reason of feeling you were stupid, and so if you feel stupid, either your reason is valid and that is evidence that you are learning, or it is invalid and that means you have nothing to worry about.

The same goes for feeling heartless. If you do something and realize it was cruel, the fact that the realization just happened, means that you weren't being intentionally cruel before, otherwise you would have felt the way you do know, while you were doing it... but you didn't, because you are more conscientious now. And it means you don't have to worry about accidently doing it again, because now you know.

Our intuition and intellect are always more powerful when combined with someone else's, and so it's impossible that we could be not worth connecting to. It is still nice to be reminded we are worth connecting to though. Our perception of life is already limited enough because we can only perceive one aspect of value at a time, and so we don't need to limit it more by adding in the bias of shame, guilt and fear.

Everything in life is seen through an emotional lens. We can choose the emotional lens we use by which aspect of a situation we fixate on. If we don't fixate on one, our intuition will pick one for us by what it sees as the most pivotal aspect of value in the situation. The emotional lens we see a situation through greatly influences what we will perceive in a situation.

Matching someone's current emotional lens shows openness to connection, because in order to share someone's experience, we have to be looking for the same thing as them to see what they see. Also, conversation goes a lot better when the snapshot of life being discussed is based on a picture from the same angle, lens, and color film is being used by the other person.

Returning to the example of gold and diamonds. Imagine one person brings up diamonds and gold in a conversation, talking about how each is uniquely brilliant, and the other person bluntly replies, "Diamonds are best! Gold will never be as strong as a diamond."

In this situation it seems silly, but that is essentially the nature of every argument, and sometimes we are the first person, and sometimes we are the second. What could have been a productive conversation, becomes a petty argument. In a more practical example: Likely we have overheard or been part of a conversation, where a story was being told, with the main focus some meaning, and someone else interrupts because they think the timeline is the most important part, and claims that the event was Tuesday not Wednesday. There are things that trigger specific emotional lenses to take over. We should become aware that the emotional lens we are using is the result of an intuitive assessment and not a trigger.

We intuitively know that the emotional lens we are seeing a situation through must match the other person's for us to see the same thing, and that is why we naturally switch to match the other person if we are open to connect. In a functional conversation each takes a turn switching to the emotion lens the other thinks is pivotal. In the most productive conversation, each emotional lens is discussed one-by-one.

Without even thinking we match posture, tone, and terminology to show our interest in seeing what someone is trying to show us. To test this, during a conversation, casually, while still engaged in the conversation, cross your arms, or if sitting down, cross your legs, and see what happens.

Animals match posture as well to show which emotional lens they are seeing a situation through. When two dogs meet often both have straight tails, then as soon as one decides the situation is friendly, he wags his tail, and the other then does the same. If one sees the situation as dangerous, their tail will go between their legs. Hair raised on their back shows they are ready to fight if it comes to that. It's not a language they are taught by their parents, it is an innate tool to help them connect, and it works—I watch my dog go and have to meet all the other dogs at the park, do we ever go somewhere and say hi to everyone there?

Most of us probably don't, at least not that we remember, I'm sure when we were very young we did, maybe three years old or so. The difference now, is that we can distract ourselves from the most pivotal aspect of value by fixating on something else, which is intuitively deceiving, because it makes the other person question themselves. We can pretend to be angry in order to ward off situations merely because we might feel awkward. We can also pretend to cry or pretend to be happy, all with ulterior motives. We weren't born knowing we could feign feeling emotions, it's something we learned watching others.

The expression of babies tend to match ours. There is a similar unspoken language we have as babies that all animals have. It is especially noted when looking surprised, eyebrows raised and eyes wide open.

The matching of emotion of babies is so consistent with all babies, that a smile returned from a baby is one of the first key psychological milestones a doctor looks for in the first few weeks.

When two dogs meet, they are looking for cues that define the situation. There are standard things that a dog if it was properly socialized as a puppy knows will return a standard response. It seems smelling the other dog's butt is a common probing test, which has three possible responses. If the dog does not allow it, they are saying that they do not want the other in their personal space, and will fight to protect it. If the dog doesn't react to it at all, then they are disinterested in playing, not because of personal space, but for some other reason. If a dog seems just a little bit embarrassed about it, but then after the first dog is done turns around and smells them, then they both want to play. I don't know that the dogs know that they are probing each other, it is probably an intuitive thing that just happens. Similarly, we intuitively probe others to see whether they are open to play or connect, and we are more aware of what response we are looking for than the way we are probing.

In general, which ways do we look for a response or indication of progress?

How we look for a response from others, is typically where conflict typically arises—if we are thinking in the artist function we are looking for something of value being added, and if the other person is responding with the engineer function by trying to take away a risk, all that will be noticed is things are not being added, and so they will think there is no response or the wrong response.

Matching emotional lenses seems to be an automatic response, that is why it is so difficult to be faked. For example. A friend starts venting, and immediately we find ourselves sympathizing, matching the tone of their voice, rhythm and even posture. Versus, instead, our boss or someone we feel obligated to please starts complaining, and we try to appear sympathetic, but find it difficult to pretend to care.

Unlike emotional lenses, functions from the systems of the psyche are not something we typically match automatically. Someone will either be looking for a response as an investment in emotion, will-power, or conversation.

The response we are looking for is an affirmative—A simple "yes" communicated or even just implied in either feeling, action or in words. If someone is looking for an intuitive or emotional "yes," then saying, "yes" with no change in affect will would mean the same as a "no" or undecided. To someone looking with the intellect, a sarcastic "yes" is the same as a real "yes." To someone looking for will-power, action is the only confirmatory "yes."

Though what we should be looking for from a conversation is a mutual increase in understanding, we sometimes just want validation that our thoughts are okay to think. We have a tendency to tell the same idea unchanged over and over again, when really if we are talking with people instead of talking at them, their feedback should influence our idea for the better, adding something good or taking away something not very good. Sure, often there is not time for more than simple answers, but in real discussions, we should notice which parts of our thought are most solid and which are least, and investigate them both.

For example, imagine a teacher, who when getting their teaching credential created lessons plans for a whole year, and then used them year after year without changing them. When year after year students in the class have the same questions, and test well in some specific areas and poorly in others, something should be done about it. A teacher shouldn't change their lesson plans radically every year, but a really good teacher, their last year teaching is the best teaching they have ever done.

"No man ever steps in the same river twice, for it's not the same river and he's not the same man." — Heraclitus

If we want to tell someone an idea and don't want them to add or take anything away from it, we should ask ourselves what our motives for saying something are. Connection won't happen if we are just talking at people instead of with them.

It seems all too often we have very vague if any expectations for the outcome of our actions and conversation. We scoff, roll our eyes, or belittle someone, and then expect that they will listen to us explain why they are wrong...

It also doesn't make sense how much we expect to come from mere implications. Even if something can be implied, there is no way that it will ever be as effective and efficient as actual communication.

Because so often implications are used instead of actual communication, essentially we are looking for anything but what could be interpreted as a "no." It can be very difficult to attune what we want to say with being careful not to offend, because people typically don't like to hear "no" and typically don't handle it well. We often go to great lengths to not have to say "no." This is why I sometimes preface a "no" with, "I know you're the type of person that can handle and prefers straight answers…" Now the "no" becomes a positive compliment to their identity showing their strength of character, and it sets a precedence of openness and honesty.

We typically don't like to hear the answer "no," but in which context the "no" comes we would rather hear is often different. Our response to "no" can range from something that spurs us on, something we don't even really notice, or something that sends us spiraling into a panic and giving up hope. The context can either be emotional, intellectual, or will-power oriented. We are not innately centered on one of the three, experience has promoted or discouraged some for specific circumstances.

Chapter 16

The three contexts we are looking for a "yes" or a "no," come from the three systems of the psyche, I have defined as, "intuition," "intellect", and "the will".

Intuition sees what is not there that should be there, intellect sees what is there that shouldn't be. Each aspect of value can and should be approached from each other these directions but intuition should go first.

Intuition decides which of seven aspects of value is most pivotal with the asset, and it suggests one of seven different actions to do, and then the intellect figures out the consequence of carrying that action out, and then the will-power brings them both together into a plan.

The fundamental actions we can make are:

1) to receive
2) to refine/dissect
3) to expand
4) to incorporate
5) to hold
6) to take
7) to give.

The Intuition is our inner artist, it sees assets or potential. What intuition perceives is not seen, heard, tasted, smelt, or can be touched, and so unlike the conscious processing of the senses which we are aware of, we cannot see what intuition is doing while it is doing it. The intuition captures a broader view of our experience, and only has to figure out which of seven aspects of value is most pivotal, which it does quickly. What aspect of value it sees, it relays to the intellect via an emotion. This emotion may not be what our attention was focused on, but something else in our surroundings that our intuition thinks is more important. This does not put intuition outside of our control—it is operating with all the self-talk we have used. The intuition is a passive approach, it resolves problems by adding a strength instead of eliminating a weakness. The intuition would be preventative medicine as opposed to the intellect which would be interventional medicine.

The intellect is our inner engineer, it sees risks or weaknesses. The intellect sees what is there that shouldn't be there. Intellect is focused on resolving what chaos it sees by using logic or order. It is the job of the intellect to debunk all the parts of the self-talk that aren't logical as they appear in our expectations. We don't consciously realize the impact of our self-talk or narration of life until the assumptions it makes build an expectation and that expectation fails.

Intellect imagines applications of logic to test the assumptions formed by intuition, and formulates expectations through seeing and extrapolating patterns. The intellect is a direct approach, resolving problems by eliminating what is weak or counterproductive.

Intuition works apart from the intellect because the difference of what they perceive. The difference between the two is so great, that if logic was visual, then value would be like sound, taste or smell.

The intuition is fundamentally nurturing, and the intellect fundamentally pruning.

As close as intuition can come to producing a visual representation of a feeling is a dream, which likely comes from the interface between the intuition and intellect.

Lastly, "the will", is our inner executive, which is the energy or determination that pulls the intuition and intellect together. "The will" has the ability to moderate between the artist and engineer functions, it is what changes the perspective of the situation. Changing perspective or the angle of the camera is a way can help the intellect and intuition connect, because while the perspective changes the correlation of the two is easier to see. "The will" puts the value of the intuition, and the logic of the intellect together into action, to facilitate contentment and composure. "The will" is what makes the integrity our character and our resilience.

Conflict can arise on either of the three systems of the psyche when either is used by itself, making the metaphorical battlefield of the conflict emotional, intellectual, or action oriented. If we bring all three functions to a situation, it is very difficult for a situation to become a conflict. If we bring only one, and someone else only brings another, conflict is almost guaranteed.

Something all three battlefields have in common, is that someone tried using an interpersonal tool, and they feel it didn't work. Like throwing a pebble up to a friend's apartment window because they won't answer their phone. When there doesn't seem to be a response, things keep escalating until there is a response or a conflict. The metaphorical pebble gets bigger and bigger until they come to the window or the window breaks.

Conflict usually starts because we want someone to do something, or someone want us to do something, and neither wants to hear "no." For example a friend asks if they could borrow something, and we know that likely they won't give it back or will break it, we want to say "no" but we don't want to hurt their feelings and risk losing their friendship. We can try to avoid situations where people will ask us for anything, or just say "yes" to everyone, but that will eventually make things worse.

I have found one of the most common causes of stress in adult life, is not being able to say "no." The fear that "no" to something asked will come across as a rejection of them can be terrifying.

The evolution of body language and self-labeling shows how much effort has been spent to try to not have to say "no" by deterring people we will likely say "no" to, and attempting to attract only the people or situations we think we will likely say want to say "yes," to. The irony of trying to have connection without conversation is the game of culture.

Why is it that hearing "no," seems like we are being attacked? Or why telling someone else "no" feels like we are attacking them?

When we feel physical pain, often we can see or pinpoint where the pain originated. Some pain has an origin we can see, like a scrapped knee, meanwhile other pain we think we can pinpoint, but it really originates in a different spot, that is called referred pain. An example of referred pain would be, pain in the right shoulder, which can be from a problem with the gallbladder. Or pain in the left arm could be pain referred from a problem with the heart. So where does pain in the psyche originate?

Mapping out the parts of our experience that can't be affected by circumstance and what can be narrows down the possibilities of where the subjective experience of pain could exist. Maybe we have heard someone say, or have said ourselves, "I just can't handle that right now! Normally it wouldn't bother me, but I'm not in a good mood right now." This leads me to believe our mood could be correlated to our pain because it is not a permanent part of us. In a machine, the higher the number of moving parts the less durable it will be, because the moving parts are where something will likely break. If pain isn't a permanent state, then maybe it doesn't have to directly do with the permanent parts of us.

It seemed very odd to me, that right after breaking both my legs, people would ask, "did it hurt?" I remember after the question came up several times, I would just answer, "No, it felt great! I was going to get up and break them again, but I couldn't because I couldn't stand with two broken legs!" Yes, I was a sarcastic and patronizing fourteen-year-old kid... sometimes. Anyway, I bring this up because I did not realize that many people in similar experiences go into shock and don't feel pain. Since then I have noticed that emotional pain is similar in the sense that it is very subjective—a whole group of us might be in the same circumstance and some are painfully miserable and others are just fine. Meanwhile, in a different situation, those who were in pain might not be anymore and those that weren't in pain might now be.

What is operating beneath or in our mood which seems to come and go?

My experience has been that sensations come and go, thoughts come and go, feelings come and go, even limbs of our body can be lost in an accident, and yet our psyche is still intact. Despite my changing thoughts, feelings and physical health. My awareness, and imagination have always been there, along with a determination.

Awareness is a process of intuition, making an association of memories of sensations to present sensations. For intuition, the more memories there are to work with, the more accurate the associations it can make with the present sensations, making us more aware. Imagination is a process of the intellect which seems to be trying to make sense of everything by considering possible consequences. The more the imagination sees, the more possibilities it can consider.

Can awareness be harmed? Well, no matter what happens to awareness, it is becoming more aware of the types of different things that happen, which is what it seems to be trying to do... so, it probably can't be harmed.

Can imagination be harmed? Well, no matter what happens to imagination, being exposed to more possibilities of ways things can be combined, and what types of synergistic effects can result, which increases the ability to consider more possibilities... so, also, it probably is not able to be hurt.

Can determination be hurt? "The will" is what pulls the awareness and imagination together, and so if both of them are tested and refined through experience, especially difficult experiences, then more refined they would be easier to pull together... so, also, "the will" probably can't be hurt.

The worse a trial or conflict is, the less likely we would have voluntarily explored that type of situation for insight. Also, the less relatable an unpleasant situation is, the less likely we would have taken the time and energy to understand the motives behind it to find out how similar they are to ours. Not that we should jump head first into danger, but when a trial comes, we can use it to learn and grow, and endure temporary pain for permanent increase in contentment and composure. Often where we learn most, is where we don't want to go.

Our memories are not stored as the actual objective things, but rather concepts of them. Any concept in our mind can be the focus of our imagination. Typically, at some point in childhood, we start drawing a line between the concepts in our mind that represent animate objects and the ones that inanimate objects. An animated concept in our mind of someone can hold the place for them while they are not present. This animated concept of them can become so animated in our mind through imagination, that even in the present of the real person the concept represents, the concept can still eclipse them.

We have likely seen examples of people in relationships with people who seem toxic for them, and they don't seem to notice it even when pointed out. We have likely also seen people doing things that they either deny doing or deny are as bad as it seems it is to everyone else. In those cases, apparently the concept of that person or thing in their mind, is a lot different than the actual person or thing.

Whether we like it or not, everyone we meet becomes a concept in our mind. The more detailed the concept of someone in our mind, the more they stick out to us. Sometimes the concept of a person is so vague that we almost completely forget about them whether or not we like them.

When there are people we don't like, it seems the more we try to get them out of our mind, the more they are there. Innately we see value in all human life, and so in order to rationalize not liking someone, we have to find a good reason. Our mind naturally doesn't see people as good or bad, it sees positive and negative potential. Because of this, as someone's negative potential increasing because of their negative behavior, that does not change their capability or potential for good. When we are mad at someone and want them out of our life and mind, to justify a permanent solution to a temporary problem, we try to claim that they don't have positive potential—that they are broken, sociopathic, or sadistic. These rationalizations don't hold up in our mind, and so we often exaggerate or convolute our claims on their hopeless state so that there is less motive and ability to debunk the claim.

I am not making an ethical claim that we are obligated to help each other even when we don't want to, I am merely stating that regardless of whether we want to associate with someone, it is futile to try to convince ourselves that they have no positive potential. What our exaggerated rationalizations do is add more complexity to the concept of them in our mind, making them stick out more.

Another futile way of entertaining hate would be to forget about people we dislike by adding more complexity to people we do like. Assumptions are what concepts are made out of, and assumptions are tested by the intellect by forming expectations based on those assumptions and watching for the results. Adding complexity to the concepts of people we want to keep in our mind would be inadvertently creating expectations they have to meet in order to stay in your mind.

It's probably best to not worry about who is a concept in our mind. As we build up reasons to forget about the concept of a person we don't want to think about, the artist function tries to add empathy towards them, and the engineer tries to take out logical fallacies we are using against them. When this happens not only is their complexity increasing, but also constantly changing, making it one of the most evolved and updated concepts. This ends up in a way defining us, because we have to either evolve in response to them, in order to keep fighting to evict them from our mind, or just accept them. The same happens with the memories or feelings that we try to pretend don't exist.

Carl Jung said, "what you resist not only persists, but will grow in size."

I would add to Carl Jung's statement, that not only does it grow, but it changes and evolves—it becomes animated on its own, even outside of our control, which makes it seem not only alive, but powerful. It's ironic, that instead of gaining understanding of other people through empathy of people who need it most, now because efforts to erase them from our mind, we have inadvertently given them Frankenstein-like life in our mind.

Reasons to hate anyone apply to everyone, even ourselves. Not to mention since we would prefer people were forgiving to us, we feel guilty for not being forgiving to others, even if it is just towards the concept of them in our mind.

The world in our mind is like a doll house, and the dolls represent actual people. The purpose is to use the dollhouse and dolls as a model to understand the actual world and people. The dolls and dollhouse can be a way of playing through complex ideas and situations with no risks, so when the actual situations come, we will see more of what is going on and what possibilities exist. With these concepts we can consider the possible outcome of both logical and value extremes, the positive and the negative—this is how we can meet the unknown and be somewhat prepared for it.

Though we can animate the dolls well enough for them to seem real, they're not.

This leads us back to the idea of mood—Both our mood and the concepts of others in our mind seem to be in our control but really aren't. One thing that seems to accompany pain is a sense of no control over the situation. Likely we all have, or seen someone, cry over something that to anyone watching seemed irrational, but to that individual, the situation carried a deeper sense of loss of control. Maybe someone blew out our candles on our cake, and though the cake was still there, and we would still eat it, and friends were still there to enjoy it with us, we cried anyway.

The irony of the dolls and the doll house, is that we sometimes think we are one of our own dolls—that we are a concept in our own mind. We try to make the doll of ourself the way we want it, but not only do others interfere, but life interferes with it. We build an identity we like, and then others criticize or deny it, or we can't rationalize well enough to ourselves how we meet the expectation of our identity. "Yes I play the guitar, but I'm not really a guitarist—I'm not really that good." Why do we make things so complicated? If someone asks us if we play the guitar, we can just say "yes." Everything doesn't have to become an identity.

It is very easy to make exaggerated positive or negative claims about ourself in our self-concept, and then have our intellect point out all the ways our self-concept is exaggerated, and have our intuition point out that we should have empathy for ourself and not feel the need to exaggerate our positive or negative potential. We don't need a self-concept, we don't need an identity, we just need to look for value and where we find it, add to it, and apply logic. Most of our happiest moments have been and will be when we are too busy doing something we see value in to think about ourselves or our identity.

I believe the root of pain is hurt pride. Pain is a debunked part of identity. Pain is a failed expectation that is being held onto.

Pride is not the only thing that makes up pain, there is threatened hope, freedom, understanding, and many other things, but if pride were gone, those things would not become pain, they would just be inanimate obstacles to overcome.

Yes, if life were specifically out to get you, and life had proved that it is bigger than you, any thoughts of hope, freedom or understanding would be futile, and we would be discouraged from even trying. Pain is when our mind tries to stop our own will-power by not giving us reasons not to try.

Chapter 17

There is something called a conformation bias, which is the tendency to look for and selectively focus on only what supports our own ideas. This is something to be weary of, but it is quite difficult to actually do.

Considering the question. "How do we unravel this tendency to animate concepts in our mind?" In my study I stumbled across an essay of one of the founding psychologists, Carl Jung. Despite a few terminology differences, it was incredible to see that we had both arrived at the same conclusion.

Here is an excerpt where Dr. Carl Jung illustrates the idea of subjective concepts of people in our mind, which he refers to as "projections."

"Up till now everybody has been convinced that the idea "my father," "my mother," etc., is nothing but a faithful reflection of the real parent, corresponding in every detail to the original, so that when someone says "my father" he means no more and no less than what his father is in reality. This is actually what he supposes he does mean, but a supposition of identity by no means brings that identity about.

"So true is this that every time he criticizes or praises... he is unconsciously hitting back at himself, thereby bringing about those psychic consequences that overtake people who habitually disparage or overpraise themselves. If, however, (he) carefully compares his reactions with reality, he stands a chance of noticing that he has miscalculated somewhere by not realizing long ago from (that person's) behaviour that the picture he has of him is a false one. But as a rule (he) is convinced that he is right, and if anybody is wrong it must be the other fellow.

"Therefore (he) thinks he has every right to feel hurt, misunderstood, and even betrayed. One can imagine how desirable it would be in such cases to dissolve the projection. And there are always optimists who believe that the golden age can be ushered in simply by telling people the right way to go. But just let them try to explain to these people that they are acting like a dog chasing its own tail. To make a person see the shortcomings of his attitude considerably more than mere "telling" is needed, for more is involved than ordinary common sense can allow. What one is up against here is the kind of fateful misunderstanding which, under ordinary conditions, remains forever inaccessible to insight. It is rather like expecting the average respectable citizen to recognize himself as a criminal."

We are learning and growing. We do not start as an evil creature and then possibly grow into being a good one; there is no reason to demonize immaturity. We all peed and pooped our pants as babies, and there is no need to loudly renounce it to save our pride, or fall on our sword and be ashamed for doing it—the simple fact is that we prefer not doing it now that we know better.

What creates resistance to positive change, is feeling that admitting we were wrong is the same as saying we are worthless. I think it is not necessary to recognize ourself as a criminal in order to change, but as very capable of criminal level actions if we are not careful. This is reason to become more aware, not more guilty or paranoid.

Life is complicated, we weren't born knowing what to do with it.

Dr. Jung said, that consciousness develops as we become aware of competing and contradictory instincts. In other words, the more problems we see, the more consciousness we have developed. Consciousness is not the whole equation, we need the strength of character to put that consciousness into action, and the conscientiousness to direct our actions in a positive way.

We are not born criminals, we are merely born unaware of the world, unexperienced with the instincts inside of us, and with no comprehension of action and consequence. Everything we learn is by either first-hand or second-hand experience. As we recognize competing instincts and try to sort them out, we learn either the hard way by first-hand experience, or the easier way by second-hand experience—either way we are learning, and that is good.

I have a friend, Dr. Gertsma who is a psychologist and has been very key in helping my sort out and test my psychological ideas with his sixty years of clinical psychology work, and his rich life experiences. Him and I enjoy playing each other in chess. I still don't know if he is messing with me by letting me win every so often. Either way, we enjoy great conversations about life while we play.

In chess when Dr. Gersma makes a move, he looks at a chess board longer than me, When considering why, I realized that he looks at the chess board longer because he sees more possible potential risks and potential opportunities. This is because he has encountered and resolved more conflicts on the board before. The better I have become at chess and the harder I look at the board, the longer he takes to make moves, and his time and energy investment seem to always beat mine. I have found the best way to balance out the difference between us enough to get at least the occasional win (if he is actually not just going easy on me...), is to add a complexity that neither of us have seen.

There are classic variations of how the game unfolds, each have a name, and each have been studied by chess masters for hundreds of years and now by computers. The closer the board gets to a classic game that Dr. Gerstma has studied, the less my chances of winning are, because I am not competing against his intellect, but the intellect of hundreds of chest masters and super computers. I am not proposing that to beat life we should be unconventional, it is very worth it to study the ideas that have preceded ours, especially ones that have worked. The good example in this case is not me, I play chess unconventionally because it is entertaining to me and Dr. Gertsma. The good example is him.

The few times a crazy idea of mine has panned out on the chessboard, it only works once on him, because he reflects on what happened, finds a solution. Then when I try it again on him, he wins. The same can be done in life.

If someone is making terrible moves on the metaphorical chess board of life, that means the complexity of the situation exceeds anything they have encountered and successfully resolved before; they are probably just moving chess pieces randomly. Therefore, the worse things a person does, the more oblivious they are to the competing instincts at play.

We notice most which particular instinct that we feel should have taken over in that particular situation, but that is only because we have seen that particular instinct successfully used in that type of situation before. Nothing in life is self-evident, all things have the pre-requisite of learning, and there is no absolute order we must learn things, so something which seems self-evident to us, may not be to someone else... yet.

Psychological maturity is the development of awareness, imagination and character. Mere age is greater not a predictor of psychological maturity.

For example, an adorable two-year old boy came running at me, and said, "Hi-yah!" right before head-butting me in the nose. Should I have done it back to him so that he knew what it felt like? No, I think we have to just accept where someone is at, and help where we can. That doesn't mean I wasn't watching him more carefully afterwards and also trying my best to explain to him why that action was not worth repeating.

Since everyone becomes a concept in our mind once we interact with them, and since we can't control completely who interacts with us, we only have two options: hope the best or hope the worst for people.

Our mind will be watching to see whether our expectation for the worst or the best actually happens to someone. It is one thing to laugh with a neighbor when he tells you he fell off a ladder. It is another thing to watch out the window hoping your neighbor climbing a ladder will fall and get seriously hurt.

If we choose to hope the worst for someone, what would that person have to do to merit us switching to hope the best for them? And what good do we hope comes from wanting something negative to happen?

In some cases, we may feel nothing will merit changing our negative hope for someone who wrongs us. The assumptions that attempt to validate the idea of an almost permanent state of criticism, once in operation, will apply to everyone... including ourselves. When we wrong ourselves it will be hard to justify still hoping the best for ourselves.

If we hope the best for people, then we are watching to see any little positive change, which will be exciting. Any positive change is reassuring because that means they will be less of the negative person that stressed us out in the first place. This also adds complexity to the way we assess value, which will apply to everyone, leading to less criticism of everyone... including ourselves.

Looking for and supporting any positive changes in ourselves or in anyone else dismantles the debilitating effects of shame, guilt and anxiety in ourselves and everyone else.

Chapter 18

There is a clear distinction between strain on the psyche, and disabling emotional pain. One makes us feel hopeless, the other excited to meet the challenge. It is what makes the difference between thinking hard and over-thinking.

Applying here the formula from earlier: there has to be a reward we want, we have to be able to see a way to do it, and have some way of gauging positive or negative response.

There are ideas however that we have no idea what to do with, ideas there is no formula to use.

For example: When someone tells us, "You should be ashamed!"

What reward is there in figuring out if that is true? The quickest way to know what reward there is, is to lie and deny the shameful thing and see what we gain. The easiest way to fix the problem is to just tell someone what they want to hear so they think we have changed. Not only does change takes time and is often difficult, but there is no way to avoid it. For example, one person might shame us for not speaking our mind and another for saying too much. That is why there is a difference between shame and a duty of prudence, shame asks for changes that are not understood, unanimously recommended, or objectively good.

How do we find out if what is being the feeling of shame is true? How do we gauge whether we are figuring it out? Anxiety, guilt, and shame are all impossible ideas that psyche lacks the tools to deal with. The reward is that maybe we won't lose connection with others if we figure out how to remove what is causing the shame.

Shame is the feeling that because of something in the past, we are unworthy of connection. Guilt is the feeling that something we are currently doing could make us unworthy of connection. Anxiety is the feeling that something we might do, or might be done to us, will make us unworthy of connection. There is a sense of duty of prudence that help us recognize things that will help us facilitate connection better with people, but that is completely separate from shame, guilt and anxiety. The duty of prudence points us in a direction and motivates us forward. Shame, guilt and anxiety spin us around and discourage us.

Feeling disoriented from our plan, disconnected from our goals, and discouraged from trying to make them happen is what produces pain—Pain is our will-power crashing into the wall of shame, guilt and fear.

This is why we just can't get over things sometimes, because we are trying to change everything except the wall preventing us from moving on. Duty of prudence attempts to fix the lack in awareness, imagination or determination. Shame, guilt and fear, attempt to fix our self-concept and identity. Awareness, imagination and determination can be improved when we find where they lack, but we do not have control over how someone sees or labels us, which means shame, guilt and anxiety can't be fixed, they can only be debunked. We don't have any control over how others label us, and we don't even have very much control on how we see or label ourselves—no one would call themselves stupid or worthless if we did.

Is our self-concept or identity something we are born with?

There is a stage in development, around the age of two, where a child refers to themselves in the third person, using whatever term someone else uses when they refer to them. I don't remember it happening to me, but the thought at some point had to have come, "apparently I'm a Michael... a you... and a he..." and then putting the ideas together to make "Michael hungry," or "Michael want."

We are typically corrected, and someone explains, what "I" is. "You should say, 'I am hungry,' or 'I want.'" We then see that to everyone else, "I" seems really important. At some point we even probably notice that the word "I" usually carries the most emotion in a conversation.

We go on a search to find this feeling of "I," others seem to have, meanwhile, we realize that we are also a "you," which also carries a lot of emotion as well. When we are referred to as "you," it seems to be an either a positive or negative label depending on our action in reference that person's ideals and taboos.

To have any hint of control over how someone sees us, we feel we have to align ourselves to be seen in reference to those ideals the way we want. It seems we can only paint the picture our ourselves in someone else's mind with the color paints and types of brushes they offer us.

Making the concept of ourself in reference to someone else's ideals and taboos is limiting, and doing it with multiple different people is even more limiting.

Though we likely know it won't work, we still feel we must paint the picture ourself before someone else does it for us. In order to control what others think, we become so busy trying not to let anyone paint us bad, that we don't have much time to think for ourselves what we want to do instead of just how we want people to see us.

The picture we paint of ourselves for everyone else with their brushes and colors ends up being different than the ones we pick for ourself. What we identify with but are scared to show to others is also its own identity, making three distinct identities in total.

Borrowing terms from Carl Jung, but defining them slightly different, I will define the concept of ourselves as an "I," as "Ego," the concept of ourselves as a "You," that we want to show to others as "Persona," and the concept of ourselves as "You," that we try not to show others as the "Shadow."

The ego, persona and the shadow are all identities, they are all just mental concepts. The ego gives us a sense of self-worth so we see value in ourselves, the persona gives us a sense of self-worth so that we can believe that others like us, and the shadow is the beast we let out to solve a problem by using shame, guilt or fear against the other person. "You don't want to see me when I'm angry," is the mantra of the shadow. The persona is the good cop, the shadow is the bad cop, and the ego is just the cop.

The Ego is an identity, protected by a set triggers, and corresponding reflexes, just as your leg kicks when the doctor strikes just below your knee. Like the tendon reflex, if it is stretched, it contracts... in other words, if the ego is attacked or even touched, it reacts.

The ego is like a home security system: the fence, the barbed wire, the gate with a code, the dogs, and everything imaginable, all set to react when a trigger is tripped. There is a saying, that "fences only keep good people out," and that applies to the ego. Though the ego is meant to be a protection to our sense of self, it only ends up being a barrier to connection. Anyone trying to connect with us, will likely be cut trying to get over the barbered wire fence, and both our security systems will be set off, and will both go into a defensive mode. The Ego is automated, and so therefore indiscriminately aggressive and hurtful.

The ego is a mass of animated primitive assumptions and expectations that are so vague that they overlap. This means one thing could have multiple different possible expectations depending on the mood, or even multiple contradictory expectations going at the same time. What immature assumptions are at play in a situation depends on which stage of awareness we are in. This is why we can get caught up in the moment and forget about ourselves, because in the last two stages of awareness, there's no room for the ego because there is no overlapping of ideas.

When identity gets involved, even a simple thing like what to do with the feeling to call a friend has overlapping ideas. Calling someone could have an influence on our identity by possibly making us look needy, nosey or controlling. It could even look like we don't trust the other person to take the initiative themselves and call us. All of these overlapping ideas compete for what is a simple answer—if you feel like you should call someone, do it. We should choose our actions by the value we see in the action, not how the action could influence our identity.

The ego was born under the strain of the shame, guilt and anxiety, which were impossible for the psyche. The ego disappears subtly as contentment and composure settle in. At that point there is no reason to identity as anything because we know we could do anything we want if we put our mind to it.

I hope this understanding how the ego was born, which is a little different for everyone, will shed some light on how to get over it. It is up to us to decide whether we treat our ego as a jester who comically points out its own flaws, or the bane of our existence.

If you made two lists not factoring in what other people think, one of specific instances or things that make you feel like you have self-worth, and one list of specific instances or things that make you feel you don't have self-worth, you would know what identities are in your ego.

If you make another two lists, but this time instances you feel others see your self-worth and instances you think they see a lack of self-worth, that will give you an idea what taboos and ideas make up the identities in your persona.

If you made a list of things you typically don't brag about because you know they are kind of messed up, but you don't really regret doing. Also adding to the list things people have accused you of doing that you deny... though not entirely accurate, it would be a good hint at what kind of things are in your shadow.

Look through all the lists and see what either contradicts itself, is not true, or out of your control. If you find anything on that list that seems to not contradict itself, is true, and in your control, consider if the action itself has value, or whether doing it proves something. With what remains, consider what the cost of doing it is.

We will end up seeing more value in life and doing more about it, if we are focused on what we want to do, and not what we want to prove. It doesn't matter who we are proving something to, it could be for someone we love, or someone we hate, or even ourself; proving is not doing. This does not mean we shouldn't feel proud of ourselves, it means we shouldn't aim for that feeling but the actual action that can produce a positive sense of self.

Some things in life bring mixed feelings, or require a big investment of time and energy before positive feels will accompany it, and we don't want to miss out on those things just because we lacked awareness, imagination or will-power.

Chapter 19

"I... love... you."

"I love you," can mean very different things depending on what love means to us, and the other person and what "I" means to both people. Sadly, and ironically, when we give reasons that we love someone, it usually is because it directly or indirectly benefits us, although we feel like when we love someone else that it is selflessly for them. If love is a gift, then a gift is only a gift when nothing is expected in return, otherwise it's a trade, establishing the condition of a deal.

"I love you because you see me for who I am," carries the implication, "If I ever feel you don't understand me, then I will stop loving you." It's not that we have to feel a profound love for someone that gives us nothing in return in order for it to actually be love, but it is a good idea to be careful that what we are saying is not implying ideas that are dangerous. Unlike love, a relationship is more like a business deal, and that's okay, because it's based on trust.

Love is a natural intuitive function, it sees assets and sees ways to support or add to it. Our significant other is not the only person in the world with assets, everyone has assets and potential, and our intuition will automatically see ways of supporting or adding. Love is the recognition of assets and potential.

Trust is different than love—our time and energy are limited, and so where we invest our time and energy is up to us, and based on where we trust the investment will go furthest. Love unbiasedly sees value wherever it is. Love is a positive hope that goes out of us in every direction to everyone. Out of vindication, to get something, or to get rid of someone else, we try to withhold our love, from some people and focus it on others. This is to either make one person we like feel more special by making our love exclusive, or make someone else we dislike feel less worthy of love.

What stops connection is the ego, both in us, and in others. The way to facilitate connection is not to try to prove we are worthy of connection, but know you are worthy of connection, and help the other person feel they are worthy of connection too.

When we feel unworthy of connection, the ego is thrusted to the center of our attention. The ego is a collection of all of our most immature assumptions, and so when it becomes the focus of our attention, we are limited to our most immature thinking and feeling. When we feel triggered, that means our ego wants to come out. The goal would be to figure out what overlapping assumptions are at play and sort them out to resolve the situation and so that it doesn't happen again. Sadly we don't always do that, sometimes we let the same things trigger us over and over again without figuring it out. If we all had a goal of learning when we get triggered things would be different, but until then, it's usually not good to trigger people.

What can we do to not set off people's reflexes?

Triggers are in the ego, which are primitive assumptions, and they are only present in the first three stages of awareness where the whole big picture is not seen. This means that if we try to point out something someone is not aware of, they will likely get triggered... because the first thing we notice about new things is the associated pain.

We have to understand that people will likely get triggered, and so try not to point out things too far out of their awareness. It is very unlikely someone will want ten different things they were oblivious to pointed out. It is unlikely someone will want anything they were oblivious to pointed out, but pointing out just one thing is a lot safer than ten, and picking that one wisely helps. Figuring out exactly which stage of awareness a person is in for a specific situation, we can then help them to the next stage. Also, we shouldn't second-guess the power of teaching by a good example instead of with direct instruction. When others see something that should trigger us and it doesn't, it's hard not to wonder why.

Something else I have realized about pointing out something to someone, is that it is a lot easier to imagine something being only five-percent a problem than ninety or a hundred percent. If someone is willing to accept some change is only five-percent, it seems like a win-win situation to change it.

For example, a politeness battle. I believe the biggest percentage of motives to go with what we think the other person wants even when they are saying they want to do what we want, is to maintain the identity of being the most selfless. Instead of saying that at least sixty percent of the politeness battles are ego-centered, we say that although possible ninety percent of it is genuine selfness, that maybe ten percent is ego-centered. This will lead to some reflection once they witness or become involved in a politeness battle, and the data will prove itself.

Another example would be, making assumptions of what people think instead of asking them. A friend wisely said, "If we love someone, they deserve more than assumptions, they deserve actual communication." So why don't we? We probably wouldn't want to hear that it is mostly because we don't trust the other person to be able to handle the truth that will come out in communication or that we think it's easier to work around someone than with them. What we probably want to hear is that we do it because when our assumptions are right, it shows how well we know someone and how much we care to put enough effort to know then. The thing is, that our motives aren't completely good or bad, they aren't even a mix of good and bad. Our motives are a mix of aware and unaware, mature and immature. I figure if you've made it this far reading so far, that I don't have to sugarcoat it, but if I were going to, I would say that "It sometimes can kind of show a little mistrust in another person when we don't say what we want to say to them."

I don't want this to be a book of suggestions but of foundational principles, but it's hard not to add them in, when I have seen them help me so much. One things that is not just an anecdote I have noticed, is the power of our personal example. We shouldn't second guess how much influence a good example can have, and there's no reason not to. Ironically, I just realized that my example contradicts itself, we are lying when we say something probably is only ten percent of the problem when we know it's at least half. How do I rectify this? I don't know. I know the principles at play are true, what to do about it, I don't know. Of course, my ideal solution is the positive logical extreme, that everyone in the world would read this book and then there wouldn't be any need to sugarcoat things... but until then, it's the best I got.

How can we be a good example, and show how to handle being triggered?

We can learn to recognize quickly when we are being triggered, and do a conscious evaluation before acting. Life seems to carry the illusion of urgency, but rarely does a situation objectively have as much urgency as it seems. For example, someone says something hurtful to us, and we reflexively want to get them back before they walk away. We don't want anyone thinking we weren't smart enough or strong enough to defend ourselves, right? And so we say something without thinking it through, and then wonder later why we did it. We just have to make a way to remember that there is nothing down the road of reflexively reacting to a trigger that we want.

In our own lives, or when dealing with other people's triggers, investing in the long term, we can avoid facilitating the strains that caused the formation of the ego, which are shame, guilt and anxiety. We can change the conversation from people's identities, to what we or they actually want to do; We can avoid absolutes and emotionally charged language, we can allow and facilitate debate of the aspects of value and logic at play in a not judgmental or accusatory way.

Only our immature parts of out intellect can entertain the idea of absolutes and impossibilities, Which means that words that imply them trigger our ego to surface. We should be careful with impossible words like: best, worst, good, bad, prettiest, ugliest, greatest, worthless, always, never, and any of the other adjectives we use to emotionally charge our ideas.

Our psyche has interpersonal tools to approach connection and conflict by focusing on learning and appreciating, instead of capturing and controlling.

Looking at the types of questions we typically ask in a casual conversation often imply we are interested to know what someone has captured or is controlling. Often the answer to "How's it going?" is "good or fine," is the same answer we would get if we asked, "how well are you controlling your life right now?" or "How is that thing you are trying to capture?" Of course it sounds odd, but we can tell that it is truth, or at least that the question engages the ego, because the answer is a state of being, which is an identity... which is the ego. Also, we can feel the difference, two people could ask the same question, but since we can feel one really means it, we sincerely answer. Reacting with the ego feels different than interacting, it feel disconnected and insincere.

"What about life have you appreciated lately?" Imagine starting off a conversation with that question.

When we ask a question, there shouldn't be a time pressure. In school we are used to being asked a question and expected to raise our hand or answer immediately. This doesn't give us the time to make any new thoughts on the matter than we previously had, and so our ideas don't improve. To really give a good response to a question, we need time to reframe it, considering it with all seven different aspects or value. If we are rushed, we normally just process it using our favorite aspect of value and then quickly spit out an answer.

If an answer immediately comes spiting up, we can be pretty certain it didn't pass through all three systems of the psyche. No situation is exactly the same, and if we approach it the same, we won't find out how it is different. We should be a little bit more aware, more imaginative and more determined every day, so really, no situation should feel the same.

Intuition processes things very quickly; that may be one of the reasons it is unconscious, because it is faster than we can make sense of while also processing everything else. After the intuitive assessment is done, the intellect still has to apply logic, then the will-power has to formulate a plan, taking the best from the intuition and intellect. Then the idea often should be assessed six more times through the other emotional lenses.

In describing the value of something, all adjectives seem to be appealing to one of seven different aspects of value. Each of those aspects of value also seems to have a specific logical criterion for the application of it, and these two things are connected. We also have seven emotions, and each emotion seem to be consistently in the context of a specific aspect of value, and corresponding application of logic.

I believe that each of the seven different emotions, is the way our intuition communicates with our conscious mind suggesting a fundamental action. When the message is received, and the general approach is handed off to the intellect for a more detailed analysis so a plan can be formed, the emotion goes away or changes to be positive. When the message is not received, then the emotion pangs louder. Each of the seven emotions is not inherently positive or negative, but is a response of the assessment of the intuition about the most pivotal aspect of value at play, and what criteria of logic should be applied.

An example, I was driving to a social gathering, one I have been to many times, and for some reason could feel my stomach twisting with fear. The associated fundamental action with that emotion is "to take," and so I tried to think of what it could apply to. I thought of several things and the feeling kept getting stronger. I got frustrated, then I realized, that although I have been to this social gathering many times, I usually don't take all the opportunities to talk to people that I should. Upon realizing that, the emotion was instantly gone. "Huh!" I thought, "Wow, that worked." Sure enough, I went, talked to a few people I otherwise wouldn't have, just to avoid going out of my comfort zone, and I was really glad I did.

Another example. I was at the checkout counter, and a person had gone into the store, got something off the shelf, and using an old receipt tried to return the item. The manager saw and came to talk to them. They kept denying it, and there was only one check out line. The manger was trying to be nice about it, and at some point the cashier let the manager keep talking to the person and opened up another lane. I felt my chest tighten up as anger set in, and I really wanted to say, "This is why all of our stuff costs more, is because they have to factor in the money they loose from people like you..." As I was finding the words to say, the feeling got a lot stronger. As I was about to speak, the anger got even stronger. My theory annoyingly came to mind. I considered the fundamental action I had attributed to anger, "to hold." "Hold myself together?" I thought. The feeling decreased. "Hold my tongue," I thought and the feeling went away. Ruminating on how annoying it was, the feeling came back. I took a deep breath, "Hold my temper," the feeling decreased. "Hold my dignity, because who am I to judge?" the feeling went away again. I thought a lot about that incident on the car ride home, and I'm glad I didn't say anything, the problem was being handled very professionally, and there I was just going to emotionally charge it by blaming and shaming.

Another example, a small child grabbed my nose. I felt the chills, which would be the emotion contempt. I had attributed the fundamental action, "to receive," and I though, "I should receive him as he was, in all his innocent awe of this world he was new to, and let him play with my nose. I made a honking noise when he pinched my nose, and witnessing the excitement it produced in him was worth whatever annoyance it might have been. The feeling didn't go away, it changed. Like the difference between rage and enthusiasm which feel very similar except one is positive and the other negative. In this situation, I felt just regular chills, I wasn't very annoyed, but I probably would have moved their hand or told them not to, but I didn't, and the feeling changed to be very positive.

This is the most pivotal part of the theory, and what should be most tested. Take the following descriptions of the aspects of value at play and the fundamental actions for each of the seven emotions, and when you feel a specific emotion, consider the aspect of value it is connected to, and how the fundamental action it is associated with, and see if the feeling either goes away or changes, and what the outcome of the approach was. The five stages of awareness, the formula of three things, and the role of ego and shame are all just to decrease the interferences of our intuition and our intellect so that the messages of our intuition can get through and be carried out.

The Emotional lenses:

1) **Contempt** is the emotion when purpose is the pivotal aspect of value. the criteria of logic to apply is functionality, determining worth vs worthless, and if the assessment is that there is worth, the fundamental action would be to receive it, and if there is not, to not receive it. The associate sense, or in other words, closest sense the emotion approximates, would be chills, or nerve fasciculations. To maintain purpose as the current emotional lens, we can give attention. Approaching a problem with this lens, means we feel the solution is something we already know and just have to apply precisely.

2) **Sadness** is the emotion when accuracy is the pivotal aspect of value. The criteria of logic to apply is reproducibility, determining reliability vs unreliability, and if the assessment is that there is reliability, the fundamental action would be to define it/isolate it, and if there isn't, to refine/dissect it. The associated sense would be sight. To maintain accuracy as the current emotional lens, we can appreciate what already is, and try to build on top of it. Approaching a problem with this lens means we feel that if we can figure out exactly what the problem is, the solution will be clear.

3) **Surprise** is the emotion when perspective is the pivotal aspect of value. The criteria of logic to apply is context, determining possibilities worth exploring vs not worth exploring, and if the assessment is that there are valuable possibilities to explore, the fundamental action would be to push/expand towards them. The associated sense is taste. To maintain perspective as the current emotional lens, we can be curious, and look forward to the freedom knowing our options gives us. Approaching a problem with this lens means the solution is not something we have already done or seen and must be explored to find.

4) **Happiness** is the emotion when connection is the pivotal aspect of value. The criteria of logic to apply is response/continuity, determining connection vs disconnection, and if the assessment is that there is connection, the fundamental action would be to incorporate it. The associated sense would be hearing. To maintain connection as the current emotional lens, we can be grateful. Approaching a problem with this lens means we feel that it is just a matter of connecting with the right person, or connecting one idea with another, or disconnecting with the wrong person or combination of ideas.

5) **Anger** is the emotion when resolve is the pivotal aspect of value. The criteria of logic to apply is resilience,

determining stability vs instability, and if the assessment is that there is something that increases stability, the fundamental action would be to retain/hold it. The associated sense would be touch. To maintain resolve as the current emotional lens, we can be enthusiastic. Approaching a problem with this lens means we feel that it is just a matter of holding our ground.

6) **Fear** is the emotion when preservation is the pivotal aspect of value. The criteria of logic to apply is security, determining danger vs safety, and if the assessment is that there is something that will bring safety, the fundamental action would be to take it. The associated sense would be stomach wrenching (butterflies in the stomach). To maintain preservation as the current emotional lens, we can empathize with others. Approaching a problem with this lens means we feel that it is just a matter of arming or taking precautions against possible threats.

7) **Disgust** is the emotion when excellence is the pivotal aspect of value. The criteria of logic to apply is transcendence, determining excellence vs degradation, and if the assessment is that there is something that helps us excel over an obstacle, the fundamental action would be to give, for example, give it more energy, or give it to others. The associated sense would be smell. To maintain excellence as the current emotional lens, we can be lighthearted. Approaching a problem with this lens means we feel that it is a matter of rising above the obstacle by pushing our previous limitations.

The Order of Interpersonal Tools in Each Emotional Lens:

There is no set order to using the emotional lenses, but there is for the tools within each lens. It is best to start with the emotional lens your emotions suggest to you, and then after that is completed, your emotions should suggest another emotional lens. The numbering system I have made for the emotional lenses is arbitrary.

1) In determining the mechanics of an operation, the first step is fairness, which is correlating responsibilities to their corresponding privileges. The second step is leadership, which is the shifting of roles and responsibilities to optimize the benefit for the team as a whole. The third step is teamwork, where we do the work partitioned out to us. When these three steps are taken, resources are outlined and allocated and order is maintained.

2) In the process of understanding, the first step is humility, which is the process of removing bias due to or against self-interest, in assessing the positive potential of things. The second step is forgiveness, which is recognition of potential. The third step is prudence, which is breaking something down into its individual components and all aspects in order to make the best judgement about it. When these three steps are taken, we unbiasedly see potential and the nature of it, which gives us the most ability to then accurately invest time and energy.

3) In finding perspective, the first step is open-mindedness, which is used to gather ideas for consideration by looking at a situation from all possible angles. The second step is creativity, which juxtaposes conclusions one by one to compare and contrast what is seen from each angle. Third step is curiosity, which is testing out the best idea that results from considering all the angles combined. When these steps are taken, we find the best angle to view each aspect of something, and the relationship between logic and value is better seen, optimizing the outcome of the next action.

4) In sympathizing, the first step is kindness, which is an investment of emotion to reach out and motivate someone. The second step is social intelligence where we consider all the possible things we could do to make a situation more enjoyable in the short and long term. The last step is love, which is action. Once we get to the third step there is no reason to question it. If our intuition already took care of the first step and our intellect confirmed it, whether or not our action also benefits us, it doesn't matter. In neither of the three steps, kindness, social intelligence or love should there be consideration for whether something also indirectly benefits us, because that is irrelevant, even if we might be criticized for it. When these steps are taken, we find the part of them that wants the best for them, and we support it, enabling the most good possible.

5) In the building the strength behind an action the first step is enthusiasm, which is strength that comes from a general grounding in objectivity. (Objectivity means that the value and logic of something can be assessed and confirmed by someone else.) The next step is honesty, which is the process of refining what is objective from what it is not by considering the nature of something. The third step is perseverance, which is holding to what we know to be true. When these steps are taken, we

maximize our ability to hold to what we have determined has logic and value because they really do have logic and value.

6) In the process of defining the cost versus benefit of a decision the first step is compassion, which is being present emotionally and defining potential assets by looking for positive claims or promises. The second step is investigation, which is substantiating possible threats attached to that positive claim, and determining how much weight it carries. The third step is acceptance, which is an agreement to the terms and conditions—it's an understanding that both foreseen and unforeseen complications may arise. When these steps are taken, we can feel confident that what we are doing won't be undermined by false assumptions.

7) In the process of building the confidence to make a leap forward, the first step is appreciation, where we look for excellence and for ways to support or augment it. The second step is humor, which is making space for solutions that are too big to process, by extrapolating past big leaps into the unknown, knowing that we can probably jump a little bit further this time. Hope then is to leap with the confidence that the leap is worth it and possible. When these steps are taken, we maximize our ability to overcome obstacles because the unknown risk becomes merely a logical next step that will likely result in success.

Chapter 20

Each emotional lens is specialized for looking for one thing. For example, the when looking for bacteria, we would use a high-power magnifying glass, and when looking at stars, we would use a telescope. There is no rule what type of lens you have to use, but I'm sure not much will be learned about bacteria with a telescope.

The picture on the cover, it was interesting separating out the colors, that even with grapes making up a big portion of the picture, the purple layer didn't actually show very much. The other odd thing was that with all the grass and leaves, that the green layer had very little on it also. If I was using the blue lens and said I saw grapes, and so you used the purple lens, you would have a hard time seeing it. It is an art, to be able to reframe a situation all seven times, and then unbiasedly overlay what we find to see it in full color.

It is difficult not to have bias towards the certain emotional lenses that seem to have worked better for us than others in the past. It is hard not to go with the feeling that we will likely get better results with the lens we are most proficient with rather than one we are not.

Here are some examples in the influence of our preference for certain emotional lenses once we have an experience where one works for us:

My friend Dr. Gertsma, when asked his earliest memory, reported that his father called him to the dining room where he had two flasks of clear liquid. He poured some of what was in one flask into the other, and it turned purple, then poured it back, and they both were clear again.

His second earliest memory was where his father was done eating, he would walk around the table several times as a sort of exercise, and he remembers crawling under the table, and feeling part of what his father was doing because his dad would see him and smile. He remembers being happy about it.

In the first memory because it was an adventure, the emotional lens represented was the surprise lens, and because of the positive nature of the experience, it likely became a preferred lens. Surprise emotional lens represents that there is something outside of the known, that would be the likely means of success. Dr. Gertsma really enjoyed high school, college, graduate school, research, and after learning Chinese and Japanese, spent time in Japan and China, and has spent much of his life exploring the mind working as a clinical psychologist and teaching at a medical school. Life has been an adventure for him.

In his second memory, the emotional lens was the happiness lens, which deals with connection. In this case he had found a way to participate with what his father was doing and noticing the subtle response of his father's openness to connection that he knew he was under the table and happy he wanted to be part of what he was doing.

Dr. Gertsma is very agreeable and interesting person, which is consistent with his earliest memories. We remember certain memories and not others, because we use them as a reference to compare and contrast new situations. I have asked many people about their earliest memories, and found that very often each memories would fall into the same category as the first two.

While being interesting and agreeable is a good thing, feeling that we are not worthy of love unless we are being agreeable or interesting is a burden to carry. My earliest memory was an adventure, and realizing that I was hypersensitive to being uninteresting helped me to debunk those thoughts and feelings when they come.

I don't want to go into what other hypersensitivities the other emotional lenses would have, because if I did, it would be theory or anecdotal data at best, and it is a personal thing for each person to learn for themselves. I don't feel bad for adding the surprise emotional lens associated hypersensitivity, because if surprise is someone's preferred lens, like me, they are going to assume the answer is yet to explore, and they will find more about it anyway themselves.

Talking with another friend, I asked her what her oldest memories was, and she said it was when she was about four-years-old, she jumped off the top of a house-boat into the water. I asked her if she enjoyed it, and she said she did, and that she climbed up and did it again, and again.

I'm sure as a four-year-old girl, standing there looking down at the water provoked several different emotions, self-preservation or fear for one. Possible anger for the thought of letting fear control her, and maybe disgust that decision was so difficult. But in the end, surprise, freedom, and adventure won out, and she jumped. The memory likely became a core assumption involved with that emotional lens. For that reason, and for the fact that the uncertainty of which emotion was most appropriate, several emotions fired, and so that memory would be several times as vivid or recallable than other memories. It is also interesting that with surprise as a preferred emotional lens, she also pursued a career in medicine like Dr. Gertsma and myself.

The next oldest memory she could recall, was early in elementary school, she was doing a quiz, and the teacher said, "time's up, pencils down. She was not done, and so hurried to finish. The teacher came over and called her by name and said, "I said pencils down." The reality that there was no fighting it was apparent. This would be the accuracy emotional lens, sadness. She said that she hated being sad, and avoided it at all costs, but every time when it seemed unavoidable, she would cry.

Talking to her about her life, it probably wasn't a coincidence that most of her accomplishments had come through a willingness to be adventurous, and explore possibilities. When things got hard, she seemed to be able to stay positive as long as the problem could be looked at as an adventure to solve, which most of the time had worked out. When it looked like the reality of the situation was unavoidable, she would break down and cry.

The sadness lens is an interesting one in the way emotion is attached to it. We cry both for seemingly very positive and negative things. The emotion of sadness, perceived as positive, or negative, are both a pull towards reality; sometimes reality is better than we thought, and sometimes it seems worse. Coming to a more accurate understanding of what is, always adds to our awareness and imagination whether or not it seems to be beneficial to our situation. It is only the ego that would rather not know what is actually going on.

Yes, the reality of the loss of a loved one is difficult, but those tears we shed at their passing, might not be the new terrible reality without them, but instead a realization of the reality of the positive impact they have made on our life, and the reality of all the possible new doors of opportunities they have opened up for us, doors that we should search out. The legacy someone we love leaves us when they die is something we are always learning more of. Sometimes we just leave it at, "I miss them so much," but what provoked that thought? Specifically what is it that you miss, and why? What did your intuition feel it appropriate to remember them in that moment?

We can't avoid certain emotions, because that would mean we would be avoiding certain aspects of value in life. When a wave of emotion hits us, our first impulse likely won't be to look deeper into it, especially if it feels unpleasant, and if the reason it was there already seems obvious. Keep searching for the meaning of emotion until it turns into a positive feeling or goes away. Also, finding the meaning of the emotion is a lot easier when we don't limit the possibilities, likely there will be something we have to change that we don't want to.

We could be resisting the emotion contempt because we don't want to pay more attention to something we already feel we aren't getting anything out of. We could be resisting the emotion sadness because to appreciate (build on) the new level of accuracy, seems pointless when everything we build on the previous level of accuracy seems to be wasted. We could be resisting the surprise emotion because we don't want to be curious about what we haven't explored yet, when we already feel there are things already around us we want to know more about. We could be resisting the happiness emotion because it is hard to feel grateful for the positive that comes from two ideas or two ideas come together when the negatives are very poignant. We could be avoiding the anger emotion because it is hard to be enthusiastic when we feel the extra energy we invest in a situation will be judged for being aggressive. We could be avoiding the fear emotion because we want to keep risks as far away as possible, and to empathize it would mean bringing the dangerous thing or person in closer. We could be avoiding the disgust emotion because it seems reckless to be lighthearted in the face of a serious situation

Chapter 21

An example of the role of emotions and how they color our experience is illustrated in an experience I had. After ordering food at a quick-serve restaurant walk-up window, I stood back to wait. Meanwhile a lady and her son came and stood by me instead of at the window. "I ordered," I told her, "thanks," she replied but didn't really move toward the window to place an order. I figured that she or her son hadn't decided what they wanted, until I noticed it appeared she had begun to ruminate; it was as if I could see a heated inter-dialog building, and finally she marched over and with her fist pounded on the window. The young girl behind the window opened the window and surprised but calmly asked, "How can I help you?"

"It should be one car, and then one person up front! I've been waiting here forever!" she screamed. "I'm sorry mam, what can I get for you?" The lady continued, "I... I just don't get it, I saw three cars get served before me!"

Anger is the emotion of resolve, or stability. Her intuition had likely suggested that the optimal fundamental action was to hold herself together and have self-control. She lost control instead of controlling herself, and not only tried to control the cashier, but control the cashier's emotions. The lady's emotion seemed to get stronger, probably because she was going the opposite direction her intuition had concluded had value, which was patience and self-control. If an emotion is the communication between our intuition and intellect, then it is suggesting a fundamental action for us to do, not for someone else to do, or us to do to them.

More to take away from this experience was, that emotionally charged, or impossible words were used, which is a good self-indicator that something we are attempting is coming from our ego, and not from our best thinking. Emotionally charged words are absolutes, for example: forever, always, never, all, worst, best, only, just, can't, or any other adjective that implies an absolute. When we use these words, it is a sign that we should figure out what we actually want to communicate, why, and what we expect to happen once we communicate it.

I have heard people say, "I just want _____ to know how much I hate them." And when asked why they want them to know that, they reply something to the effect that it will make them feel better to have vindication. I personally don't typically feel better after trying to control what someone else thinks or feels, and less likely if what I wanted them to think was negative.

In the case of the lady ordering food, the process of interpersonal communication was backwards. Our intuition assesses value, communicates it to our intellect via an emotion. A value assessment doesn't have words or even definitive symbols, and it is the job of the intellect to put it into something logical which can be explained with words or diagrams. Those words or diagrams once shared with someone else, in reverse can be understood by their intellect, and started through their own assessment of value and application of logic. After making an intuitive assessment of value, and then turning it into words or diagrams, it can be communicated back to us.

If your appeal to objectivity is near enough to objectivity, their value assessment should be the same or better, and so there is no reason to project emotions. Projecting emotions is the attempt to by-pass someone's assessment of value.

The lady had a whole conversation with the concept in her own mind of the girl behind the counter, and by the time the actual girl had a chance to participate in the conversation, the conversation was over. Instead of a conversation, the only thing communicated was the emotion she projected.

Why did the lady become so upset?

If three cars in the drive-through were served before her, the ego would say that it proves that the person working the window thinks she is three times less important. The lady wasn't expecting her ego to be challenged, she just wanted food. She was pleasant with me, because I was not attacking her ego. Maybe some shame, fear or guilt someone else was using against her was on her mind, and because she was struggling to fight it, the ego was already out dealing with it. Once the ego is already out, it is much easier to be triggered; she just reflexively reacted.

When we thoughtlessly react, we lose the opportunity to meaningfully interact.

The lingering sense of shame, guilt and anxiety we carry from other conflicts can keep us close to a trigger point as often as we carry it.

The ego has a counterfeit version of value, which is selflessness, and a counterfeit version of logic, which is capability—both are relative to other people and are something that has to be proved.

To prove our identity as selfless we have to be relatively more selfless than everyone else, meaning we give more than we get. For example, sometimes out of the blue, someone does something nice for us, and our ego says, "Great! Now we are relatively less selfless than them! Relatively more worthless!" Instantly we want to do something to set the balance back, by doing something nicer for them.

How could something like a spontaneous act of kindness trigger us? In the victim stage, all we see is pain, and so we find pain everywhere, either the gift was not exactly what we wanted, when we wanted it, or how we wanted it given to us. In the fighter stage we have to protect our identity as selfless by not letting others be more selfless than us. Even in the creator stage we feel that we have what it takes to prove we are more selfless by giving something better.

A gift is only a gift if nothing is expected in return, otherwise it is trading, or bartering. We should give gifts, and also allow others to give gifts.

The way we talk about ourselves or others is often in reference to identity and likely how that identity is selfless or capable. This means when we are given a gift, we tend to not focus on the gift, but what it implies about the identity of the giver or ourself. For example, if you are at work, and you need a pencil, and you ask if anyone has one, and the co-worker that most annoys you offers a pencil, would you take it?

"I don't need a pencil that bad..." would probably be the thought or even the vocalized reply. It's just a pencil though, right? Why is it more than that?

Cognitive behavioral therapy says that we attach meaning to situations, and when there is a distortion in how we attribute meaning, it causes unpleasant feelings. A possible meaning that could get attached to the gesture of accepting the pencil, would be that we are no longer annoyed with them and accept them; maybe we feel we aren't ready to do that, because we think merely offering a pencil doesn't mean they will stop doing what annoys us. Another meaning that likely would be attached to the situation, is that they would think we owe them a favor, and we don't want to feel like we owe them anything, because we don't want them to forget that they owe us more than we owe them, or don't want to give them the power to make us feel guilty, or shame us later when they demand too much of us and we don't comply.

I think we spend too much time trying to apply meanings to what other people do, and not enough time trying to find meaningful things to do. Are we really content hating a co-worker year after year? Even not considering the benefit to anyone else, the reasons to try to move past the feelings of hate is worth it for us. What would be the point in holding onto hate?

If someone annoy us, we are probably not the only ones annoyed by them, and so if we can get them to stop by making them feel bad until they do, we will be doing everyone else a favor right?

If that were the only option, maybe... but though we are likely not the only one that is annoyed by them, it's not possible that everyone is. And even if we have personally gone and talked to ever single co-worker and asked them if that person was annoying and they agreed, why do we think shaming, guilting, or scaring them into changing will work?

When we try to fix other people, we get to feel we are right and they are wrong. What are we supposed to feel when we realize that we are wrong? That we do the same thing we criticize in others?

If we look to point the finger at someone that is doing something worse than we are to distract ourselves from feeling the need to change, we should expect others do the same. We have to show that we are willing to look at our own faults, and that will show a good example that it's not as scary as it might seem.

We should be like the chemist Roy Plunkett, and be willing to cut our mistakes open to see what is there. If we do, we might find something new, like he found Teflon.

Our self-talk gets stored as memories with implied assumptions, those assumptions form expectations, and failed expectations held onto produces emotional pain. It is up to us to screen our self-talk for implications which are unproductive or false. We should be careful of self-talk involving identities, even ones that seem good; the better sounding an assumption is, the more likely we are to try to hold onto it even when it fails.

It is a big assumption that how we see ourselves or how others see us is how we actually are. This false assumption leads us to trying to prove that it's true. Proving is a never-ending battle; the identity of being selflessness, because it is relative to others it is subjective, and always open to be discredited.

The endeavor to prove selflessness becomes more and more ridiculous as proving selflessness becomes a game of who can expand the distance further between their contribution to others, and their contribution to us.

For example: we do something that benefits us a little and the other person more, and then they turn around and do something back that benefits us more and doesn't benefit them at all. So, what do we do? We do something better back to them, that actually comes at a sacrifice to us. Finally, we can't figure out a way to make the benefit gap bigger, or don't have the energy to do it, and we start to feel shame, guilt or anxiety. The easiest mitigation at that point for the ego is self-sabotage, because loosing means winning in the game of selflessness.

The ego has no sense of ridiculousness, it will just keep trying to prove the impossible/ironic until it is completely exhausted. When our intuition carries the assumption that our ability to connect is at stake, as long as the assumption remains that we must be selfless to be worthy of love, then it will keep doing the ironic and ridiculous.

The other part of the ego wants to prove capability, which conveniently is opposite of selflessness. It is also relative to others, and the goal is still to increase the gap between us and others. In this case, it is for us to gain more, and them gain less. This game also gets pushed to the point of irony, where for us to prove we win, we not only have to gain more, we have to gain everything and even sometimes have the other person lose something.

If our ego wants to identify as being capable, then everything becomes a competition, even things we have no control over.

A funny example of this is when someone told me that they were a "good pooper." I thought that was a pretty odd thing to brag about or identify as; it didn't seem significant enough to be harmful, but it was. This person said that recently they were in a hurry, but their bowels weren't, and although they figured they should probably just wait and not rush things, their ego being trigger that one of its identities was at stake yelled, "But I'm normally a good pooper!" The idea of losing part of its identity caused a reflex, and they pushed so hard, they ended up a couple weeks later getting hemorrhoids. I don't know if it was a series of trips to the bathroom where their pooping identity was in jeopardy or not, but it happened. Anything in the ego will eventually have negative consequences.

In the pooping identity crisis, the body is what suffered. Attempting to prove capability usually comes at someone else's expense, it leads to the easiest mitigation, to sabotage them.

To prove selflessness, we end up sabotaging ourself, and to prove capability we end up sabotaging others…

This begs the questions: Can a self be selfless? Can we be capable and not be the best at something?

Why would we want to be selfless, unless it benefitted us in some way? It is not possible to do something positive for someone else that does not also have positive repercussions on us as well. The opposite is true, it is impossible to do something positive for yourself and not have it also benefit others.

For example, if I invest time and effort in being more stable, who does it help most?

I don't know, it's impossible to say—daily someone will benefit from more stability in their own life, but also people can learn stability faster watching them, or lean on them when they need support. So, an investment for one person in stability or any other aspect of value is neither selfless nor selfish, it just has objective value, just as much objective value as if anyone else did it.

"(Humility is) a state of mind in which (you) could design the best (building) in the world, and know it to be the best, and rejoice in the fact, without being any more or otherwise glad at having done it than (you) would be if it had been done by another. (Humility) in the end, (leads us) to be so free from any bias in (our) own favor that (we) can rejoice in (our) own talents as frankly and gratefully as in (our) neighbor's talents—or in a sunrise, an elephant, or a waterfall." -C.S. Lewis

Being a self, we cannot be selfless, but we can be humble, and unbiasedly add value wherever we can. Anything an individual does because they see value in it, doesn't just benefit them, it benefits everyone.

The ego gets in the way of everything of actual value or logic.

The ego only sees comparative value, and cannot distinguish itself from the paper it writes on, the car it drives or house it sits in. The ego is looking for the sense of "I" -ness that others seemed to have when the idea of "I" was first introduced to us. "I" seemed to carry such authority and excitement. "I" seemed to be a declaration of what someone had control over. It is no wonder one of the first words a child learns is, "no." "No" is one of the first senses of control we have.

Control is not an aspect of value. The ego does things just for the sense of control. The assumption is that "I" is only distinct from its environment if "I" controls it, otherwise "I" is just a part of the environment. The ego therefore doesn't like feeling controlled.

The idea that we can ride on a train together, and still be distinct from each other and distinct from the train doesn't make sense to the ego, it will still find a way to prove it is separate. Since the ego just wants the feeling of control, all it has to do to achieve that feeling is maybe by being in the best seat, or even just sitting higher than everyone else, or maybe even just talking as if they own the train.

Looking through a friend's childhood pictures, I noticed that in every group picture, candid or not, their head was higher than everyone else's, and there were too many pictures for it to be coincidence. That was a very consistent trend in many other aspects of that person's life. If the ego can accept "pooping quickly" as something to use to prove relative superiority, then being the top of any picture makes just as much sense. If we are not careful, the ego will use other people as the means to prove its own power.

We should probably try to understand people and life before we try to control them. We might find trying to control life or people changes us more than them, and not in a good way. Resisting the urge to change people gives us the chance to find out that people can be loveable without even changing them.

Chapter 22

The ego is not an infection or inner-monster, it is a transition stage as we figure out life. Every day we are learning, and processing all the information, and make assumptions about things. We start off with very immature or primitive assumptions, like, "all vegetables are bad," and then we realize we like asparagus, and corn on the cob. Maybe we even start to understand the vitamins and nutrients at play, and how to put certain foods and spices together to improve the flavor. Now if someone asks me if I want a salad, I ask what kind of salad it is, instead of assuming because there are vegetables in it that I won't like it.

Our assumptions start off very vague, often very false, and for the most part useless. As our assumptions get better, they become more concise, accurate and useful, and there is no limit to how much they will improve.

In calculus, instead of saying that two plus two equals four, it is said that as a number approaches exactly two, is added to another number that approaches exactly two, the sum approaches exactly four. It may seem like it is adding unneeded complexity for just plain numbers, but as the complexity in a formula increases, the need for complexity of the numbers in that formula also increases. If the number two was a measurement of distance, if one person was measuring with 2.001 and the other with 2.01, and both calling it 2, there would be an increasing discrepancy in their answers the further an equation using them is expanded.

In math there is a concept called significant figures, which says that an equation's accuracy is limited to the level of the least accurate measurement.

Combining these two ideas: In some equations it is necessary to divide by zero, or divide by infinity, both of which are impossible to do. Something interesting happens however in those equations as the very small number that is still more than zero, or the very large number that still is less than infinity, approaches zero or infinity—it starts to approach an answer.

For example: if I asked what you would do if I gave you ten dollars, it would change if I asked what you would do if I gave you a million dollars. Things might change if I asked what you would do with a billion dollars, and maybe even change again with a trillion dollars. But at some point, the increase in money would make no difference, because you would run out of ideas to use the money for. What you would do with more money than you could ever spend is probably the same as what you would do with an infinite amount of money. That is calculus in a nut shell.

Just as ideas can be taken to their logical extreme, and intuitive feelings can be taken to their value extreme. We can start with imperfect, biased or subjective ideas and feelings, and taking things to their logical and value extreme, we will start to see a trend that approaches reality or objectivity.

Also, as the complexity of our assumptions increase, the possible complexity of expectations can increase.

In math, there is a type of equation called an iteration, which allows you to solve an unknown variable by substituting into the variable any value, and then working the equation through to get an answer. The answer that comes out is now the new variable. This new variable can be used to work the equation through again, producing a newer variable. After several iterations of the equation, the new variable when input in the equation comes out the same—that is when you know you found the correct unknown variable.

Optimization of assumptions and expectations works like an iteration, it doesn't matter much what your first guess of the variable is, running the equation enough times will get you to the answer. Guarded assumptions and expectations stops the iterative process, and leaves us with an immature guess for a variable.

When there is an inner or interpersonal conflict, we can ask, what aspect of value is most pivotal in that instance. Then reframe the situation using a different aspect of value, and see what improvement there is, and what costs are at stake. Then we can again reframe the situation with another aspect of value, until we have pictured it in all seven different contexts. Each time we assess the situation with a different emotional lens we gain more insight. There is no limit to how many times we can assess something, but to avoid over-thinking, we should test the assumption in some way directly or indirectly before assessing it again.

For example, a typical assumption and expectation for teenage years, "If someone kisses me, that means they love me, and if they love me, that means I am worth loving, which means I have worth, so... if I can get someone to kiss me, I will feel valuable, and if I feel valuable, I am allowed to be happy, otherwise I should feel sad as motivation to do what is necessary to become worth being loved."

...that is a long series of assumptions, with a lot of variables... and it is, but it happens all too often.

Algebra tells us that we cannot solve more than one variable with one equation. Science tells us to test one thing at a time. English teaches about logical fallacies. There are many tools we can use to recognize long chains of vague assumptions like this one, with large gaps in both value and logic. Because the last assumption in the series of the example has to do with self-worth, it would seem, that to throw out any part of it, you would be throwing out your self-worth. This is why we often struggle and to try to keep the whole chain of misled expectations... till heartbreak shatters the whole chain of assumptions.

If I asked right now, "what is one of your assumptions you should challenge?" what would you say?

If I asked you: "when was the last time you felt, shame, guilt or anxiety, and what assumptions were involved?" If I asked which of those assumptions you should challenge, it would be a lot easier to point one out.

We can follow the unpleasant feelings to see where the primitive assumptions are hiding. Without an ego, it would not be possible to experience shame, guilt or anxiety, and once it is gone, those feelings will go with it. There is a saying, "the squeaky wheel gets the grease," and in the case of our primitive assumptions, once we grease them all, not only will they stop squeaking, but we will roll with less resistance.

Each good assumption in a situation makes it easier to build another good assumption on top of it which allows us to comprehend more complex ideas, which allow us to handle more complex situations. This is how we get real momentum in life, it's not through self-esteem. Confidence that our assumption is good doesn't mean it is; what makes an assumption good is that it is concise, accurate and useful.

The reason assumptions have to be made, tested and remade over and over again, is because we don't know how important the components that make it up are until we know what those components do, and we won't know what they do until we can use them. This is why it is a process of trying and stumbling into how to use something better, and then understanding how it works a little better, making it easier to use it better.

When we are young we often value things based on pretty arbitrary factors like color or shape. Color and shape are factors, but very rarely the most important factors, although buying something merely because it is our favorite color, likely helped us realize it wasn't as important as we thought, which helps us make a better decision the next time. It is very natural to want to feel heard, seen or valued, but like our favorite color, it is rarely the most important factor, and we shouldn't let it be the only factor we base things on.

The comfort of feeling heard, seen or valued is enjoyable, but not reliable for seeing things how they really are. Feeling comfortable has nothing to whether there is a real reason to be comfortable, for example, any parent knows when their young children are quite, it's because they are likely getting into trouble... "It's so nice to have the house calm and quite," isn't worth saying, because your three-year old toddler is quietly destroying the bathroom or kitchen. I don't mean that is a pessimistic way, obvious it is possible for kids to be quite and not mischievous—what I mean, is when kids are quite, it isn't a guarantee they are not being mischievous. All German Shepherds are dogs, but not all dogs are German Shepherds.

"Comfort is the one thing you cannot get by looking for it. If you look for truth, you may find comfort in the end: if you look for comfort you will not get either comfort or truth—only soft soap and wishful thinking to begin with and, in the end, despair." –C.S. Lewis

There are ways to trick ourselves into feeling heard, seen and valued, but we should be saying things worth listening to, do things worth watching, and increase value, whether or not anyone but us ever listens, watching or values it. We are here to develop ourselves, not our egos.

Would it be possible to never develop an ego?

Maybe in a sense we could grow up without ever having an animated or personified ego, but the primitive assumptions which make up an ego would still be there until we improved them. The difference in whether we look at the sense of self as an inanimate object or not, only changes how it feels to challenge those assumptions. The difference between a sense of self and an animated ego, is that the animated ego squirms and screams when it is challenged. An inanimate sense of self when it is challenged, quietly disappears like the night turning to day.

What started the ego was a desire for a sense of "I"ness. What starts to undo the ego is a desire for a sense of togetherness, which must turn into desire for togetherness without worrying about the feeling of togetherness. The ego is an identity, and when we focus on it, we look at other people in order to see how they see us. Once we stop focusing on our identity, we can look at others to actually see them. When we look at other people to see them, we see them for who they are instead of whether they make a flattering mirror or not.

The ego started developing early in life when we likely identified as preferring something simple, like a certain color. We could pick blue for instance, as a way to define ourself as being with someone else we like that also likes blue. We also could pick it because we want to distinguish ourself as separate from someone we don't like. All the ego has to process is, "Is this blue? If yes embrace it, if no, push it away."

It is not to long after that, we likely start identifying with more complex things, like super heroes and sports teams. Typically, about high school age, we have maybe three to five things we identify with. Funny, kind, motocross racer, for example. Likely we have chosen at least one identity to prove our selflessness, one to prove our capability, and one to connect the two or to prove our will power.

When we focused on our identity, our perception of life is essentially reduced to a question of which of the few categories something falls under that we identify as, whether it is positive or negative, and how negative or positive. This attitude puts everything in reference to us, making things seem negative just because they don't fit into our arbitrary identity. If I would have stuck with the things circumstance happened to show me hade value, humor, kindness and motocross, I never would have found music, writing, medicine, psychology and everything else.

Chapter 23

If there were only one dimension to life, only one aspect of value, then decisions could be easy and definitive. With seven aspects of value or dimensions to life, definitive solutions are not possible. This is why in the heat of the moment when we only see one aspect, and try to solve it, then afterward thinking about it more we sometimes change our mind. Often it is not that we changed our mind completely, but found a different aspect of value that is more pivotal in the situation than the one we use first. If two aspects of value both seem pivotal but produce a different conclusion, we end up switching back and forth.

Looking at school through the surprise lens for example, school could seem a lot more like prison than an adventure, and if it is only one of those two extremes it could be, then we will be frantically trying to escape one moment when it seems like a prison, and excitedly learning the next when it seems like an adventure. For another person, through the happiness lens which aspect of value is connection, high school could be seen as the best place for opportunities to make and stay connected with friends or the most dangerous place for drama.

What we hope for is often seen through just one emotional lens, partly because we have our favorite emotional lens, and partly because adding a second emotional lens usually reveals some side-effects of the exciting prospect.

For example, the adventure lens might excitedly say, "Wow, I've never eaten a whole gallon of ice cream before, what a fun adventure." Or through the resolve lens, "I wonder if I have enough resolve to finish a whole gallon of ice cream." Meanwhile adding the accuracy lens might suggest possible health consequences that override whatever positives are seen in other lenses.

We don't have to try to solve every situation before it happens, it's nice when we can figure out how to approach a situation before it approaches us first, but it's hard to know what to prepare for until it has at least happened once. Theories can't be built on other theories unless they are tested. Big theories with big consequences should be tested indirectly first before acting on them. There are some things that the consequences outweigh what we will learn from testing it, methamphetamines for example, definitely not worth trying once. After seeing several patients with complete heart failure who were only thirty years old because of meth-use was enough indirect evidence for me to not want to try it.

I drank a whole gallon of water one time, because I was thirsty and also trying to prove my resolve or something... I don't know, I didn't really think it through very well. After drinking it, every time I moved I could feel the water move inside me, and pain as things inside me stretched to attempt to hold the stomach full of water in place. I do not need to eat a gallon of ice cream now to figure out whether it has value, I can just build on my water experience to make the assumption that there is at least one valid reason why it would not be worth it... not to mention the shock that much sugar and fat would have on my pancreas.

Sometimes we don't even realize what assumptions we are testing, but still can benefit from recognizing the failed expectation when it happens. When we feel a negative sensation, we can ask, "In this situation, what was I expecting to happen? And why?" If we start to feel anxiety, guilt or shame, when we begin to examine our expectations, we can figure out why the ego was trying to guard them. If the thought of challenging an assumption feels like death, then we can be pretty certain that our focus was on our ego.

Once you can feel no pain in challenging an assumption or expectation, and instead feel excited to see what revised assumptions and expectations will produce, you can be pretty sure you are close to seeing the big picture of life. Until then, we should always look into what bothers us.

If apathy, hostility or resentment arise, a helpful question to ask is: "Am I trying to control something?"

Or better, "Would my current problem be gone if I could just control something or someone else?" Then follow up that question with questions like, "What is the connection between that person and my problem?" and, "what are all the possible ways this problem could be fixed that don't involve that person?"

Where we will likely find the most about ourselves and what we can change to understand and enjoy life more, is exploring what triggers us.

Before the ego comes out we feel the trigger get tripped, and it is a conscious choice then to let the beast out to take care of business.

There is a reason why some assumptions haven't gotten challenged yet, and that is because they seem to work really well sometimes. If the assumption that when we throw a tantrum seems to have worked ever since we were three-years-old, it might seem like a viable option when we don't like our service at a restaurant, or a family member or friend won't do what we want. But of course, throwing a tantrum only seems like a good idea in the heat of the moment when the impulse begs it. After thinking something through rationally, it would be difficult to conclude that a tantrum is the best interpersonal tool to use.

The ego seems separate from us, because the primitive assumptions it is made of, overlap with more refined assumptions we also have, and so the ego can suggest things our better judgment wouldn't actually want to do. The primitive assumptions would be there whether we animated or personified them or not, that is, until we refine them. The ego feeds on itself; it makes poor decisions, that we realize later we wouldn't have done, which sends us into a panic that we can't trust ourselves, and in the panic we often let the beast out again.

When we ask ourselves why we did something, we should actually figure out why instead of just beat ourselves up. When we find that we lied to someone because we didn't want them to reject us, then the next time we are scared we might be rejected, we can remember that lying didn't help last time.

If we let them, shame will prevent us from reflecting back on previous experience, anxiety will make us fear new experience, and guilt will distract us from our present experience. The past, present and future hold a treasure of knowledge, and we will find that treasure when we focus on the experience and our impact on it, and not the impact of the experience on the image of us.

Chapter 24

At any given moment we are either feeling, thinking, or doing something. These go in an order, first we are intuitively feeling the assessment of value, deliberate what logic applies in order to carry it out, and then we do the action. Everyone else is also in one of those processes. Connection happen when we are assessing the same instance of value. Then together we can deliberating on what logic applies, and lastly, when we are both invest time and energy into it.

If we don't care to see what someone else sees, connection can't happen. The first step in connection is to recognize that other people also have the capability to find value. The second is to realize that logic is universal. Third that efforts can be combined for better results.

It is just a matter of bringing our assumptions close enough to objective reality that they corelate with someone else.

Sometimes we are deliberating, and hoping that someone else will join us. However, discussion can't be started until the pivotal aspect of value we have found is assessed by the other person and they see the same aspect of value. Once we explain what asset we see, the value assessment can be done by the other person, and then they will be able to join us in the deliberation phase. If they don't seem to be engaged in the deliberation, it might be because they are not there yet.

Similarly, sometimes we already have something we want to do, and the other person hasn't assessed the value, or deliberated out how to apply logic to it yet, and so they don't seem to be eager to join us in the action phase.

When we force someone to do something with us before they've found actual objective value in it, and applied objective logic to it, then they are merely just playing along letting us puppet them. To avoid that, we must trust our own ability to find objective value and apply objective logic, and then naturally others will join us there... eventually.

Chapter 25

Interpersonal tools help us connect our intuition to our intellect, and work to connect us to other people.

The ego has counterfeits of interpersonal tools, which is just using the wrong tool for the job, making them weapons instead of tools. When we approach a situation with the wrong tool, it won't work, and so as we keep trying to force the tool to work, it becomes a weapon.

For example, when warning someone crossing the street that a car is coming, being assertive and yelling for them to watch out would be appropriate. Patience in that context would not convey the warning in time before the accident had occurred. However, when someone isn't paying attention to you, screaming at them to get their attention would not be appropriate.

There is a tool for each of the seven emotional lenses combined with each of the three systems of the psyche, making twenty-one in total. Like-wise there is also a weapon for each of the twenty-one tools.

The tools/weapons of intuition are:
1) Fairness/Exploitation, 2) Forgiveness/Obligation, 3) Open-mindedness/Intolerance, 4) Kindness/pseudo-altruism, 5) Enthusiasm/Rage, 6) compassion/Provoke pity, and 7) Appreciation/Complaining.

The tools/weapons of the will are:
1) Teamwork/Leeching, 2) Prudence/Fanaticism, 3) Curiosity/Pride, 4) Love/Bartering, 5) Perseverance/Relentlessness, 6) Acceptance/Competitiveness, and 7) Hope/Skepticism.

The tools/weapons of the intellect are:
1) Leadership/Manipulation, 2) Humility/Intrusiveness, 3) Creativity/Uncreativity, 4) Social intelligence/Exclusion, 5) Honesty/deceit, 6) Investigation/Ego inflation, 7) Humor/Dogmatization.

The line between an interpersonal tool and a weapon is blurred, and each person has to make the journey on their own of discovering the how and when to employ each tool. This can be done by having clear definitions for each. The definitions I gave in the preface are merely a starting point. Because intuition can't be described in words like the intellect can, words can only convey half the picture at best. Each tool should be considered in relation to it's opposing weapon, and a journal could be made to record the outcome when the definition is tested.

In a general sense, a big difference between a tool and a weapon is what we are trying to control. We cannot control other people, we can only facilitate someone else seeing the same instance of value.

We shouldn't treat other people as if their ability to see value depends on us, and we shouldn't have our ability to see value depend on someone else.

In the process of thinking, after a value assessment and a logical application, there is an internal confirmation that the process was done correct. We shouldn't depend on others for our own internal validation, but concerning interpersonal affairs, validation is necessary. In communication on a radio, after a message is finished the person says "over," and the other person receiving the message says "ten-four."

The trick is to figure out which of the three different channels the radio to say "ten-four" on; respond by investing emotion, opening discussion, or investing time/energy in the form of action, or just all three to be safe.

Intuition cannot be expressed in words and so a hug is one of the better forms of intuitive interpersonal communication. A hug means that we want to be present with someone because we appreciate them, and we support them. We shouldn't worry if there are things we can't express. We shouldn't be scared of silence. If someone is open for communication, taking time to find a way to communicate something shouldn't trigger them. We shouldn't assume it will, that wouldn't be trusting them. If silence does trigger them, they probably don't want to have been triggered it, and will be glad for the experience will help them work through it.

Love is not something we must try hard to do, love comes naturally, it is trusting that love is enough—that is the hard thing to do.

We can help love be enough by becoming proficient with all twenty-one interpersonal tools, and not using any weapons. We could probably look at the list of interpersonal tools and weapons ourselves, and immediately identify several tools we use regularly, and probably several weapons we use regularly as well. After a thorough investigation of it, we could see the role each tool and weapon plays in our life. It's just a matter of identifying the weapons we are using, and swapping them for the appropriate tool.

The first key of connection is to eliminate the ego, which blocks all connection. The second key after that, is to respond in whichever of the three systems of the psyche they are looking for a response.

For example: When a parent is focusing on seeing compliance in a child, as the child struggles to resolve his or her will/autonomy against the parent's, the child might try emotionally investing to see how they can earn the opportunity for more autonomy. If that doesn't work, they might try emotionally withdrawing. If the parent doesn't respond to that, the child might continue withdrawing more and more until it is noticed. By the time the parent notices, the parent thinks the problem has nothing to do with them, because no matter what they try the child stays emotionally withdrawn. We carry the last major conflict with us, either to try to figure it out, or to try to prove our point. In this case, now the child is trying to prove a point that they were hurt.

When a favorite tool doesn't work, it is often forced until it becomes a weapon. If that still doesn't work, the favorite weapon comes out, and then when the favorite weapon doesn't work, a weapon we are less familiar with comes out. Then with the increasing panic and the lessening familiarity using others weapons, the chaos and damage become worse. When that desperate attempt doesn't work, the most drastic weapons at the most drastic levels come out. Full panic hits, complete chaos breaks out when the last resort weapon is used, and everyone gets burnt.

So how do we let someone know if we think something they are doing doesn't have value?

If they are focused on their ego, that is the problem why value doesn't seem to be present. Helping someone not feel their self-worth is at stake, and to facilitate someone to put the focus back onto actual aspects of value will get them out of their ego.

A conflict does not end the possibility of connection. Yes, there can be a conflict, that someone can turn the wound to their pride into a trigger to protect themselves from it happening again. And yes, that trigger while around them will likely send them into their ego quicker than it would have before, but just as we don't like our selves sometimes and eventually get over it, someone can't stay in their ego forever.

The better we become at using interpersonal tools, when someone does come out of their ego, odds are better this time we will connect. And the better we become at not using interpersonal tools, the less likely we are to trigger someone again.

The ability to connect with others is like the ability to make a garden of an empty field, it will become what we make of it. From intuition seeds of value are planted in the intuition, and nurtured by the intellect, and blossom into the will. The closer we are to someone else, the less we can distinguish what we or they have planted, and both just unbiasedly nurture it. When both are planting and watering, it makes twice as many seeds able to be planted, and twice as much nurturing to plant, and likely twice as much fruit from each plant.

A connection is not limited to two people, in fact, we are either connected to everyone through the objective value and logic which is assessable to all, or we are alone in our ego. We are either gardeners in the collective garden of life, or not.

Chapter 26

New concepts have to be rooted in something we already understand, and so before we can start building a concept, we have to figure out where to attach it. We have to make space and lay the foundation for ideas. For example: Physics wouldn't make much sense if there wasn't a foundation of math first.

It is a constant task of laying foundations and making space for what ideas will fill them. We don't know what we don't know. When we find something solid, it makes sense that other ideas will likely be able to build on top of it, and when there is an empty space, that there is probably something that fills it. We watch as our assumptions are challenged, and the immature ones fail and are reassessed, and the ones that hold move forward to the next level of testing.

We shouldn't beat ourselves up for having used interpersonal weapons instead of tools, we all want connection, but don't always go about it the right way. It's not because we are intentionally choosing a bad way, we just don't always know what way to go. Sometimes we try to avoid having to use a tool in the moment it was needed because we feel taboo using it, or incompetent with it, and then the job gets harder.

For example: I was at the gym and walking between occupied benches, trying not to bump into anyone's barbells while they were lifting. Just as I was stepping over some weight plates on the ground, I felt my foot make contact with something, and heard something tumble across the floor. I looked down to see a cellphone tumble and the come to rest on the floor.

It seemed odd for a phone to be in an isle way, and I looked around to see who the owner might be. To my left I saw someone standing on their head with their shirt off flexing their back muscles. I pieced together what had happened, the phone had been propped up on the side of a weight plate on the ground to record video or pictures, and though I had noticed the plate while walking I hadn't notice the phone. I quickly tried to set up the phone where it probably was, but it slid back down. I realized in order to pick it up, I would likely end up being filmed. I knew it probably already at some point showed me picking it up, and I felt embarrassed. I left it filming the ceiling and hurried away.

I watched from across the gym, and saw the guy pick up the phone. I could see he was confused because it wasn't propped up like he had it. He started looking through the footage, and I realized that not only had I messed up his video, but now I had also wasted his time. I should have just been like, "Hey bro, sorry, I accidently knocked over your phone," and he could have immediately restarted his project, and just deleted the old one.

A gamble in avoiding conflict ironically, is often the birth place or catalyst of conflict. We try to run away from one conflict and run head on into another.

The interpersonal tool of honesty could have been used to tell him what had happen, but I used a weapon instead and escaped. Honesty can be met with conflict by the other person, but us not using weapons reinforces the habit of using interpersonal tools instead, and although the conflict may still have been similar, at least you are not reinforcing sub-optimal habits and you are giving the opportunity for connection to happen instead of conflict.

When someone else use weapons, that doesn't change what has objective value and logic—it's not a valid excuse to say the other person started it. There can be objective value and logic in physical personal defense, but not in using interpersonal weapons.

Our ego stores what it sees be successful to use later. Using interpersonal weapons reinforces the effectiveness of weapons in our own mind, and in the minds of people around us. Trying to resolve one conflict through our ego which was started by someone else's ego, will only produce more ego in everyone directly or indirectly involved.

We have a drive towards interaction with people, but until we challenge and refine our primitive assumptions, instead of connection, it will only be our ego clashing and reacting with people's ego.

"Life doesn't make any sense without interdependence. We need each other, and the sooner we learn that, the better for us all." --Erik Erikson

Connection doesn't mean letting someone control your emotions, will, or intellect, it means that you understand that someone is capable of learning and appreciating value and logic the same as you. Maybe not to the same level of complexity in the same things, but that they are at least not broken.

Chapter 27

Assumptions in the intuition work like a seed being planted, that then at some point, suddenly a plant coming out of the ground. Before the plant breaks the surface, roots have already gone into the ground. In the case of the intuition, the seed whether well thought through or not, was dropped by the intellect through self-talk, and roots form before the stem breaks the ground.

It would be difficult to map out the roots of a plant without pulling it out of the ground, but that doesn't mean knowing exactly where the roots go in intuition is important. Each seed has general root patterns, and that will help placement and spacing of plants, the rest is not as important. Similarly, with interpersonal connection, because intuition is involved, it is not an exact science... but it doesn't need to be. Here are some directions finding a solution could go through, that might be helpful.

First idea: **2-minute rule**

When speaking, we should allow for the other person to give some sort of response at least every two minutes or so, giving them the opportunity to add to the conversation and potentially influence its direction. If someone is really listening, they will likely have at least clarifying questions, to make sure they are follow the whole train of thought, or an epiphany that your inspired that they are excited to share. If what you are saying is novel information, then those ideas will need space for those ideas to be received, and that takes time—the speaker can facilitate space for ideas their ideas to be placed, but not perfectly. If the information is not novel information, it doesn't need to have space made for it, but it also doesn't need to be said, or at least doesn't need to be belabored.

It is really difficult to go more than two minutes without responding, and so if we have attempted to connect for more than two minutes, and have not gotten feedback, then we are either looking for the wrong type of response, or not giving them opportunity to respond.

Yes, allowing for input could steer the conversation in a different direction than the one you wanted, but a conversation is not one person imposing a monologue on someone else, it is synergy of ideas.

If the conversation is engaging, it will have produced an idea in the other person's mind, and if they don't get a chance to share it, they will have to choose between trying to remember it at the expense of hearing the rest of what is said, or just abandoning their thought in order to keep listening to you. This decision means they would have to decide the purpose of the conversation, to make you feel heard and valued, or actually listen and add value.

When something we are saying inspires an idea for someone else, the surprise emotional lens is what is typically used because it is something new. Eyes widening and eyebrows lifting are good signs to give them a chance to say something.

Second idea: **1-10/10 scale.**

We are accustomed to answering questions with a "yes" or a "no," although a complete yes or no might not be accurate, and it doesn't leave the conversation open to add context. "Yes, but I would rather _____," works, but not always do we know in the moment what we would rather have, or whether we want it very much more than the original option.

When the importance behind asking something is measured in an absolute "yes" or "no," and we feel pretty neutral about it, communicating that neutral sentiment into an absolute "yes" or "no" either we will feel needy, like we are calling in a huge favor, or feel disconnected from someone because we are scared to ask them for a favor.

As an intermediate between "yes" and "no," "kind of" is useful, but in many contexts, it just comes across as a passive aggressive way of saying "yes" or "no" without actually saying it. This may seem philosophical, but it has significant impact on interpersonal relationships.

Consciously or not, we typically keep track of the relative number of things we ask for compared to what others ask from us. We unconsciously do it as a way to measure our own selflessness or capability and theirs. Is someone who asks more things of others selfish or incapable of doing things on their own? That's the question it seems to imply.

For example: someone asks us if we need help, and we think it would be enjoyable to have their company, but don't want them to feel obligated to help, what do we say?

Probably, "No it's fine. I got it, but thanks." This happens so often, that offering help and not expecting to actually help is a social convention of its own. It seems like a win-win, because the person offering looks selfless for offering, and capable to be able to help, and the other person looks selfless for not making the other person help, and looks capable to be able to do it by themselves. Great, now we have proved we are worthy of connection, by not working together... or being honest... or connecting. What would show selflessness and capability would be sincerely communicating with someone else.

If we try only asking one thing for every two things a friend asks of us, in order to not feel selfish, the other person wouldn't be able to also do the same. They likely at some point not want to feel selfish for asking twice as much of us as we do of them. It may seem some people don't mind asking double or triple what we ask of them, but part of that may be because they know we want to feel selfless, and if we complain about it but still do it, then we do feel selfless. That's half of the nature of co-dependency.

So maybe we try to keep asking favors even. We decide we don't want to ask anything unless it is very important, and if they do the same. Then at some point we just avoid asking anything at all, even if it's important, and become bitter about it.

A possible solution is the number system. We are asked what we want to eat, and we say, "six out of ten a burger," and as long as we trust each other, the other person could say, "eight out of ten I want tacos," and we get tacos.

Adult life seems plagued by not wanting to say "no," which puts us in a lose-lose situation, this system could solve part of that.

C.S. Lewis writing about common conflicts that arise with the guise of selflessness: "If each side had been frankly contending for its own real wish, they would all have kept within the bounds of reason and courtesy; but just because the contention is reversed and each side is fighting the other side's battle, all the bitterness which really flows from thwarted self-righteousness and obstinacy and from the accumulated grudges of the last ten years is concealed from them by the nominal or official "Unselfishness" of what they are doing or, at least, held to be excused by it."

It is a much greater sign of love, to feel free to speak your mind and ask your wishes than for someone to guess or assume them. When we are too scared to speak our mind, it is not out of love, it is out of a lack of trust and self-confidence.

People we love deserve more than implications drawn from ordinary mannerisms as a form of communication. Those we love deserve the engagement of our best faculties to express ourselves, our greatest energy employed in paying attention, and as open as we can make our heart for change. There is no reason to leave a conversation with anyone unchanged by them for the better, and less reason to leave a conversation with a loved one the same as we were before talking with them.

Third idea: **Speak People's Language**

It often surprises me the difference between what other people remember about the same experience compared to me. As we develop interpersonal tools, the order of development can vary greatly; we can by chance develop several tools in various different emotional lenses under the same system of the psyche. This means we are more capable of perceiving and dealing with value, logic or action in those situations. We naturally try to notice and remember the variables that correspond to the tools we are most proficient with incase we might end up needing them later. We remember best what pertains to the tools we want to use most, because we can make the most use of them.

For example, someone might be wondering whether we remember our last conversation together? And if we not only remember the conversation, but have thought about it since, and have more to add, they would likely be excited.

Or, maybe someone might be wondering whether we remember the last place we went together? If we not only remember, but have ideas to discuss of where we can go next, they would probably be excited.

Or, if we remember the last emotional experience we shared with them, and what it was about?

Do we remember the last accomplishment done together?

On the flip side, do we remember the last time someone emotionally, physically or intellectually withdrew? If that is the case, they probably feel ashamed for using emotion, will or intellect as a weapon, but if the solution to the lack of connection is still unknown, it is very difficult to let go of what has now become a conflict. It is not a matter of proving that the conflict has been resolved, but understanding that the ego has probably set triggers in that area, and investing in the development of that corresponding interpersonal tool will likely be beneficial.

A connection journal of instances of synergy and instances of conflict could be a good idea to know what someone is more sensitive about. Once we know, it will be easier to facilitate more synergy, and avoid conflict.

Fourth idea: **Remember what you have concluded you should remember.**

A journal of connections or conflicts. Writing or diagramming out purpose and effect of interpersonal tools and weapons. Or a list of questions that pull you out of your ego by making you really think. Maybe writing a life statement would be helpful. Then edit or rewrite it whenever you feel your direction in life seems vague or off.

Something that I have resolved to remember, is not to try to do two contradictory things. Which means I have to check what I want to do to make sure it isn't contradictory. I have to consider my long-term and short-term goals, because it is usually a conflict between them.

Once I have decided on a course of action, I shouldn't at the same time imply or do the other. For example: be patient while also letting the other person know indirectly that they are testing my patience.

An example of a question that has helped me pull my focus off my ego is:

"Am I moving toward value and logic, or away from possible conflict?"

Running away from conflict will lead us wherever seems most safe from conflict, which is wherever, and with whatever we feel we have the most control of. A pursuit of value and logic will lead us to see value and logic in more places, with more ability to add to it, and less desire to try to control it.

Value can't be control, it just is, and we can learn from it or add to it, but we can't change it. Only the ego thinks that things have to be captured and controlled for them to have value.

Another question, "Am I being compliant just to not have to figure out what I think, in order just to avoid conflict, or because I really think it?" Or, "am I being rebellious to be vindictive, hostile or am I actually being authentic?"

At a pretty young age, we find ourselves struggling to keep our head above the water against imposed ideals and taboos. There is a destructive idea that our ability to connect depends on the mastery of other people's ideals and the complete avoidance of their taboos. Because the easiest measurement of connection is compliance, we are labeled as either good when we are completely compliant to someone, or bad when we are not.

In the classroom, the playground or at home, complying with nine out of ten things is still likely considered non-compliant; it seems to be all or nothing game, either we are the golden child / star student, or the rebel. It is at such a young age we are expected to choose which role we want to be.

Several times I have seen small children trip and fall, then look at their parents to know how they should feel about it. In each case, the emotion started off the same, it was confusion, but not panic, and then depending on how the parents reacted, the child's emotion would change. "How do my parents, friends, or critics feel about this?" is a much different question than "how do I authentically feel and think about it?"

When we are 100% compliant or 100% rebellious, it is very unlikely that it was our own assessment of value and application of logic that lead us to the exact same or exact opposite conclusion as someone else. We shouldn't be different just to be different, but we also shouldn't let life by-pass our mind or emotions either. Life has its own logical consequences, we don't need to impose extra ones on others, it just confuses things.

Fifth idea: **Work with the most amenable resource**

Emotion, time/energy, and intellect are all resources, and we have each developed differently the ability to manage each of those resources. For busy people, despite already having many things on their list of things to do that all take time, penciling in time might still be a lot easier than figuring out what to do with emotion. We might have figurative trucks and tractors to manage large amounts of intellectual material, but only have a picnic basket to carry our energy or emotion. So, when interacting with someone, it is wise to figure out what resource they feel most comfortable working with, and working with that resource.

This is the same for the emotional lenses. A person with happiness as their favorite emotional lens can handle a lot of connecting, but someone with connection as their least preferred lens might not be able to handle as much. Someone with fear as their preferred emotional lens might be okay planning something out thoroughly, but a person with surprise as their preferred emotional lens might get anxious having things set in stone. If we take the time to figure out what resource someone is most comfortable handling, working together will go a lot smoother.

It is interesting how we typically enjoy being helpful, and when a friend asks for help, it actually feels nice to be needed, or be wanted, but yet we often don't ask for help when should. Part of that is the ego, that has something to prove, but also it just might be from passed experience of being rejected. Our confidence to trust that people are willing to help us, will increase as we increase our ability to work with whichever resource and through whichever lens necessary.

Sixth idea: **Being authentic over being polite**

The idea of politeness can be helpful but can also be detrimental. Politeness guarantees a certain amount of kind things said, but doesn't guarantee any will be sincere.

It's hard to know what we don't know, and so it's nice that friendship exists, because since we all learn things in different orders, we can share what our awareness has found, or what our imagination has come up with. This process is natural, but taboos have been created around anything that might offend someone. The most common way around offending someone when we want to say something that could be taken offensively, is giving a compliment before giving constructive criticism. I think though well intended, it conditions us when we hear a compliment, to expect some kind of criticism. Compliments should be spontaneous, not forced.

Two common sentiments I have felt in myself, and see quite often in others, is when a compliment comes, the question seems to be, "What are they going to ask me for or criticize me of, now that they have paved the way with a compliment." This ends up being a fairly strong barrier to trust and actual validation.

A saying stuck with me from early in my life, "people are like banks, as long as you have made more deposits than withdraws, you can make pretty big withdraws."

I have taken that assumption through many iterations and tests, and have metaphorically broken the bank with people quite a few times. In most cases I wasn't making a withdraw for myself, but for them or for the connection between us. What I have come up with, is "I shouldn't try to manage them or the whole connection between us myself, when I could just ask them if they would like some insight I have realized and let them decide."

Most of the time the answer to whether they want the insight I have found is "yes." Sometimes I follow the question with asking how much of an answer they want, and surprisingly enough, most of the time people just tell me to give it to them straight. The critical part of this whole process is not so much finding the perfect timing or words, although best words and timing help, what matters is whether someone trusts you. The way we make deposits in the bank of friendship is trying our best to do what is in their interest, and then they will trust we want the best for them. It is difficult to not notice and factor into our opinion what someone does that irritates us, or what they don't do that would benefit us if they did, and so we have to factor ourselves out of the equation while considering whether we should offer a criticism. I have noticed an interesting look that people give me when I offer a criticism that has nothing to do with me, that doesn't even make me look smart for pointing out. And that expression usually signifies they will consider it.

Similarly, "I love you, but I just don't trust you," is an odd but somewhat common phrase, and the times I have heard it expressed to others, or received it myself, it wasn't accepted well.

When we just want to complain, but don't really want to change anything, we know which people to talk to. When we really want to change, we know the people we should ask. It's kind of hard to swallow, because life can create quite a lot of strain, and it doesn't make sense to add more strain by being told or figuring out we need to change, but if we do need to change, we probably should. The ego will lead us to finding someone to tell us we are completely alright, so we can "rest," even we know we are not—that is probably a sub-optimal approach.

Intuition sees value and wants to increase it, but can't actually do it without applying logic. Betrayal by a friend tends to be harder to deal with than by anyone else. But can a friend actually betray someone?

I think friendship is born when two people are at the co-creator assumption level of the same principle. That shared principle can vary in impact on life. The principle could be entertainment, or community investment, or anything else, and though often one shared assumption at the co-creator level leads to more, there is no obligation for that to be the case.

I think there is a principle of loyalty which is pivotal to friendship, and if each person is at the co-creator stage on that principle, that friendship will likely be solid. Both with my actions and also sometimes in words, I make an effort to let friends know, that I know that they don't intend to hurt people, and that if I find myself hurt, I promise not to assume it was intentional. Also, if there is something to bring up about it, I trust they will see value in working it out.

I have found that most incidents don't even need to be brought up, because just as I have awareness and imagination that is continually optimizing, so does everyone else. I try not to impose my timeline and agenda of change on other people.

I have a puppy, and I was playing fetch with him, and he stopped, and I called him to come, and he didn't, and was shocked how quickly it triggered me for him not to listen... then he started pooping. I quickly realized how controlling I was being, and how much that same sort of attitude taints my other relationships.

Sometimes the other person might not be listening to us, and they don't have what we think a good excuse is, but then again, we are fooling ourselves if we think we always have the ultimate best motives and actions, and the only valid excuses.

If what is meant by love or friendship is enjoying someone's company, we wouldn't always have loved ourselves or been our own friend. If we want to connect with someone, and share our awareness, imagination and will-power, it would probably help to share the same benefit-of-the-doubt we have for ourselves with them.

"We judge ourselves by our intentions. And others by their actions." – Stephen Covey

We should make judgments but not pass judgments. Likely the difference between someone else's intentions and actions are maybe easier to see, but just because of that, they shouldn't be more harshly judged. The feeling of irritation might be our intuition pointing out in someone else what we should change ourselves—I know for myself that has very often been the case.

If we are looking at others in order to better look in ourselves then that judgement is great. If we are looking in ourselves to understand others, that judgement is also is great.

Seventh idea: **Love beyond the surface level**

We should appreciate other people's success, and help where we can, but it's not our job to "fix people." Sometimes pointing out someone's failure in order to help them, might be a step towards objectivity, but it also might be a distraction from a bigger step towards objectivity, that they would have made on their own.

We all have the ability to see value and apply logic, being a friend means understanding that, and supporting the other person in that process instead of taking that process over. If we try to "fix people," we can get distracted in feeling that other people's failures are our failures, instead of seeking success by being an example that through our ability to challenge our own assumptions, we can see value and optimize it.

One thing that often haunts us from our personal history, is wishing we could go back in time and fix relationships we feel we couldn't fix then. This wish can lead us to repeat the same sort of sub-optimal relationship situation, in order to prove that now we have to power to fix what we couldn't fix before. "Fixing" a significant other as an adult in a way you couldn't fix a parent, sibling or friend as a child is a sub-optimal reason to enter a relationship. Yes, hopefully we have learned, but our experience should help us help others, not be a ball and chain we carry the rest of our life, pushing us towards dysfunctional relationships.

In order to help someone else without making it about us, we can be mindful, and when we see someone disappointed, we can ask why. In order to learn we first have to ask a question, and when we see someone that looks disappointed, they probably have a question on their mind they don't feel they could answer on their own.

I have found that a typical mentality we have toward who and when we want to open up to people, is when someone cares enough to really notice what's going on. When asked how someone is, my experience has been I get one of three answers: "I'm okay/good/doing great/tired."

I started asking when someone replies, "tired", "tired of what... or who?" and I usually get an odd look, like, "Are you reading my mind?" and then they openly tell me what or who they are tired of, and seem to really appreciate that I really cared enough to figure out that the surface level answer was not the whole picture. The same could be applied to the other answers, "Okay with what?" "Good enough for what?" or "What kind of great?" Or my favorite, when I see someone that looks frustrated or down, I ask them if it's their birthday. They usually give me a really weird look, "No... why?" then I reply, "You just look so happy." And I try to say it with a straight face. They usually end up laughing, not sure at first if I'm crazy or they are. "I really didn't think I was smiling," they reply. "Why not?" I ask, and then they typically open up.

When we try to promote conversation instead of force compliance, we will find agreement instead of resistance. I have also found that in the process of promoting any idea, instead of bartering, a gift of extending trust before it is proved is better, and often empowering.

Eighth Idea: **Don't serve food cold**

All too often when someone does something that bothers us, we take along time to think about it. Then once we come to a conclusion we present our conclusion already all thought out and expect the other person to be able to process what took us a week in a matter of minutes. Getting something "off our chest" doesn't have to be one big vindicating event, if we don't know someone well enough to guess fairly accurately how they will handle something we tell them, we probably shouldn't just dump it on them, especially if we are doing it just because we think we will feel better about it.

Thoughts and feelings about a relationship should be discussed by both people in the relationship so they can process it together. Yes, independently one can realize a relationship is not right for them, and in that case, there is no reason to talk about anything. A relationship should make life easier not harder, and no one should stay with someone that causes them fear. If a person tries to process things together as they come with someone else, it will be pretty clear pretty quick whether or not the other person can or wants to work together. If they don't, then the relationship won't make it far enough for the end of the relationship to be a big deal.

There are two options to discussing conflicts. The first being, to think it out and then present it at a speed and in a way the other person can process. This is the best one when we are really not sure what we are thinking or feeling, and are pretty sure what is triggering us has very little or nothing to do with the other person.

The second option is to let the other person know, that you have a thought that you would like to talk through together instead of trying to come to a definitive conclusion by yourself. If this is the case, then pick the most important part of the thought or feeling, and share that. This isn't to be cryptic, but to make room for an almost completely new way of looking at it. This can be difficult, because we are pretty sensitive to guilt, and if someone we care about brings something up, hear the whole message and change if we need to. If we think about it and the only things we can think of that would solve the conflict have to do with the other person changing, then we should probably think it out first and then share it. If both people could change, or if you want help figuring out more clearly a vague feeling about something you should change about yourself, then yes, talk it through.

This takes an agreement, that both trust the each other won't hide things—that there is no reason to pry, because there is nothing else to find. That anything withheld is because it is uncertain and/or unimportant. It might seem odd to hear a very specific idea and not assume there is anything attached to it, but it should be understood, "anything else attached to this idea is so uncertain that I have no preference towards it, in fact I want it to be replaced by something better, which is why I am presenting it."

The more we mature, the more things we will feel we can talk about in the moment, because we it won't be simply a matter of us not getting triggered. The conversation will be more about a better connection than less conflict.

Ninth Idea: **8 second hug**

Yes, eight seconds is a long time, and no, I am not recommending giving everyone an eight second hug. The shell we put up or mask we hide behind is made up of what we think logically think will keep us emotionally safe. Intuition is not fooled by shells or masks, intuition which is non-verbal communication bypasses whatever façade we put up, so that hearts can connect. This makes us feel vulnerable, because we can't hide out hopes and fears from being seen from other people's intuition. We may not remember the last time we felt an overwhelming feeling of belonging, but likely it was when we were the most vulnerable; like being held as a newly born infant, not aware that we were naked, and nothing we could do about it even if we did know, being held tightly in someone's arms who completely loved us.

It may not have been a parent or grandparent holding the newborn us, but if it wasn't, for sure it was the nurse there at the delivery, responding to our cry to be held. We resist the one thing that allows someone into our life—vulnerability, by cutting off the intuitions communication which is non-verbal. We often avoid eye contact, avoid letting people see us cry, and avoid allowing ourselves to be held.

I wish I had known earlier in life, what C.S. Lewis put so well in his book The Four Loves, "There is no safe investment. To love at all is to be vulnerable. Love anything and your heart will be wrung and possibly broken. If you want to make sure of keeping it intact you must give it to no one, not even an animal. Wrap it carefully round with hobbies and little luxuries; avoid all entanglements. Lock it up safe in the casket or coffin of your selfishness. But in that casket, safe, dark, motionless, airless, it will change. It will not be broken; it will become unbreakable, impenetrable, irredeemable. To love is to be vulnerable."

We live in a world of alphas, where we all want to prove we are worthy to be held by proving we can hold ourselves. When we hug what is said intuitively is, "I will hold your pieces together so you don't have to worry about falling apart. Take a rest in my arms for a moment and remember that you are loved."

When we hug someone, at about eight seconds on average there is a deeper breath in and then an exhale as our body actually relaxes. You can definitely feel it, we are rigid, and then we melt. Don't count while you are hugging, but if it is longer than about eight seconds before the other person relaxes, then they are really stressed out, and scared everything will crumble if they relax. If it is less than about five seconds, that means something else, not something consistent enough to be able to diagnose similar to taking longer to relax. You'll just actually have to communicate and figure it out with the person.

This is where "soft science" meets hard science. Cortisol is a stress hormone, it is made to reallocate energy in the body to what is vital when all the energy possible needs to be put towards something difficult. This mean things like the immune system, making neural connections for things like short term memory, and maintaining the high energy state of REM in the sleep cycle are all minimized. This means it is easier to get sick, we forget things, and don't sleep well.

What else does cortisol do? It makes blood vessels more sensitive to hormones that regulate blood pressure—this is so that it can respond quicker in pumping blood. It also increases adrenaline, which increases the heart rate and blood pressure, but also helps us focus and stimulates the release of endorphins, which numb pain and produce euphoria. Because of this, it is possible to remain in a stressed state for a long time, and still be very productive, but it's not sustainable. Cortisol also interacts with insulin and produces weight gain, and all that high blood pressure with a high heart rate wears out the heart faster.

If you held your arm straight out in front of you, after a minute it would start to burn, and eventually you couldn't hold it up any longer. When we are using a muscle but not moving it, it is harder for the muscle to get rid of the lactic acid that builds up. We all hold our stress in different parts of our body, most people either hold stress in their neck or back. There is some muscle we don't realize we tense, but do to keep our body in alert mode so it keeps pumping cortisol. At least once a day we should give someone a real hug so that at least for one second of that day, they can just relax. Relaxing the muscles is good, but a hug does more than just that, I can't say for certain the exact neural pathway that is involved, but whatever the "belonging circuit" ends up being in our brain, it lights up and calms the cortisol driven alert mode.

The non-verbal communication of a hug or eye contact should precede the verbal communication of words. I would venture a bet that most marriages struggling don't meet each other after work with at least an eight second hug before they ask how their day was. We shouldn't expect words to be able to describe emotions, especially when we can just look someone in the eyes and then hug them and feel their emotion for ourselves. The part of hugging that is the best, is after we relax and allow ourselves to be loved, and so if our hugs with those we really love aren't at least eight seconds, we are totally missing out.

In closing:

Socrates said at the end of his life, "…the greatest good for man is this: every day to conduct conversations about 'the irretrievable' and about the other things about which you all hear me discussing and questioning of myself and others; the unexamined life is not worth living."

The word irretrievable in Greek contains the derivative of the word 'virtue" and I would translate it as "objectivity," because though objectivity exists, it is just impossible with the subjective perspective we have to grasp or retrieve absolutely. Through iterations of making and challenging assumptions we can reach functional or near objectivity. When we each challenge our own assumptions, and then discuss together what we find, we chart a course to objective value and logic, and there we can objectively meet.

It is our choice to react or interact with life. Life is more enjoyable when we spend our energy figuring out what we really want to do, instead of what we want other people to do or what we think others want us to prove. If we think we will be able to stop reacting to life only as soon as we can make life not give us reason to react, we will probably be too busy fighting life and everyone in it, to actual enjoy it.

We shouldn't be scared not to have an answer, but be excited to find one, and determined to then find a better one after that. Hopefully everything we did yesterday is at least a little sub-optimal because we are a little better today.

We will know we have actually found a real answer when it spawns a chain of new questions.

If we really focus on life instead of ruminating on our sense of self, which feels riddled with shame, guilt and fear, every day we will find more value and see more logic than the day before. Every day we will be a little better, and have a little more contentment and composure, until that is what we always feel.

The unexamined life is not living. The concept of "I" is the only thing separating us from the reality of "us." Don't let what the ego imagines as intermediaries or means to connection be what stops you from actually connecting. We don't have to find a reason why we are worth connecting to, we just are, and looking for a logical reason for an intuitive asset blinds us from seeing it. Everyone wants to hold a baby, and a baby doesn't have any special skill to offer.

We are all more similar than we think, for one, we are all inhabiting the same world, even if it doesn't seem like it.

An irony of life is that somehow we have gotten fixated on our sense of self, when what we really want is a sense of belonging. We exist whether we have a sense of existence, and we belong whether we feel it or not. Not only is there enough space for everyone, but a void is left if we are missing anyone.

What gives us a sense of self often has very little to do with us and more to do with the culture or time we happen to be born into. The feeling that accompanies letting go of our sense of self might really be the sensation of shedding the bias we didn't know we had.

"No one, not even a genius, can entirely step out of his time, that despite his keenness of vision his thinking is in many ways bound to be influenced by the mentality of his time"
-- Karen Horney

We may not be able to step out entirely of the mentality of our time, but if there was one aspect of it that we should step out of first, it would be the focus on our sense of self.

Kellen Heller said, "Self-culture has been loudly and boastfully proclaimed as sufficient for all our ideals of perfection. But if we listen to the best men and women everywhere ... they will say that science may have found a cure for most evils; but it has found no remedy for the worst of them all—the apathy of human beings."

Abandoning our fascination with our sense of self may seem like death, but really it will be the birth of something new. No permanent part of ourself is bad, it is the temporary parts, that we can grow out of that can seem to spoil the whole thing sometimes.

Aleksandr Solzhenitsyn in The Gulag Archipelago said, "If only it were all so simple! If only there were evil people somewhere insidiously committing evil deeds, and it were necessary only to separate them from the rest of us and destroy them. But the line dividing good and evil cuts through the heart of every human being. And who is willing to destroy a piece of his own heart?"

To step out of the influence of our era, and to step outside of the insecurities that undermine our innate ability to see value, will be like completely cutting out our sense of self as we know it. This might feel like cutting out a piece of our own heart, or even losing the whole thing, but like a phoenix it will be reborn, but now reborn outside of the influence of our era and insecurities we were born into. We were born into a culture and taught to value certain things and not value others, whether or not they have intrinsic value or logic. The family or culture we were born into doesn't not have to be our fate, our mind is more powerful and complex then the precedence and circumstance of society or the calamity of tragedy and opposition.

Whatever work we put into figuring out society and culture will be lost as society and culture change with the times. Whatever work we put into finding value and understanding logic cannot be taken from us.

The question is not "what does the sum of what I have done mean of my self-worth?" but rather, "What meaning from all that I have already done, can I use to make more meaning of the opportunities that surround me?"

"The richest and fullest lives attempt to achieve an inner balance between three realms: work, love and play." --Erik Erikson

Work happens when "the will" is not hindered by guilt. Love happens when we let the intuition see what could be there without being blinded by shame. Play is what happens when we let the intellect toss around ideas and shake out the parts not worth keeping, without being frozen by fear or anxiety.

We have two choices in life: make the focus of our life a fight for our survival against death and pain, or make finding and adding to value in life our focus, which will let love into our life and allow us to thrive.

Aristotle said, "It is the mark of an educated mind to be able to entertain a thought without accepting it."

I would say that the mark of a heart full of empathy is one that can hold the assumption of value based only on another person's claim, until they can see what the other person sees. That doesn't mean doing what the other person does, but leaving space for their claim to be true at least until we can see why they would claim it. It is being able to be present with someone despite preconceived notions.

Yes, we have likely seen enough of life to know to be careful, but that doesn't mean we should live in fear. We have seen enough to know that life can be wonderful, and we have experienced enough to know that seeing and making the world wonderful depends on us.

"The mind is not a vessel to be filled but a fire to be kindled." – Plutarch

The laws of nature are impersonal, and if we do nothing life will either destroy us or define us, but if we take life seriously, life will strengthen us as we figure out how to operate in it.

"It is not enough to have a good mind; the main thing is to use it well." – Rene Descartes

It is easy to enter every moment of a day so burdened down as we try to carry all of our hopes and fears for that day, that we miss the good in every moment. Every moment is worth investing a full moment in.

How we approach every moment matters. Shakespeare said in <u>Antony and Cleopatra</u>, "Give me my robe. Put on my crown. I have immortal longings in me." Our innermost longing is not merely to survive, but to thrive, and we share that longing with everyone else.

Connection comes most intimately from looking for that innermost longing in others and ourselves. Love says, as Jordan Peterson wrote, "I want the best, for what wants the best in you." We ought to love ourselves and want the best for what wants the best in us. There is a longing inside to love without reserve or limits and allow ourselves to be loved with ultimate vulnerability.

We are more than what we can hide behind a mask, and there is no reason we should try to hide it. We are not the chemical mess we feel like at times, we are amazing—we defy the law of the universe that says all things trend towards chaos and emptiness.

Walt Whitman said, "I am not contained between my hat and my boots." We are not contained between our fears and our past experiences either.

We are born with awareness, imagination and will-power, and combined with any other awareness, imagination and will-power both will be increased; that is the value of connecting. What we are born with is all we have or need to give. You were born worthy of connection, don't ever second guess it!

Yes, it may be dangerous to open up and let people into our life, but it is fatal to attempt to keep people out. Choose love, choose to see the goodness in life unbiasedly wherever it may be, and choose to make life better for yourself and everyone, whether or not anyone else wants to help.

It is very normal and understandable to want to feel heard, seen and appreciated; at some point however, we have to make the decision to say what most merits hearing, do what is most worth seeing, and give what is most worth appreciating, whether or not anyone sees, hears or appreciates it. There is a saying that "integrity is how you act when you think no one is looking." I say that moral character is what we do despite all that would sway us otherwise, whether that be potential for fame or fear of insignificance.

"No positive effort is so small that good things won't come from it, so do it!"

Intro to Systemology of self:
A study of Anatomy of Mind and Emotion—AME

Life doesn't look like life when drawn in one dimension when there are really seven quite distinct aspects to life. Likewise, we have three functions to operate in life, and for them to work properly, they must be used, and used in order. Whenever just one function is used without the other two, instead of seeing assets, identifying risks and making a plan, it is not a complete action, and won't be productive.

The general concept of pathology, is that the intuition, intellect, or will-power reflexively tries to operate alone, typically through only one particular emotional lens, and without hardly any thought put into it. It does this to avoid taboos on interpersonal weapons, that have become so sensitive that the corresponding tool is almost completely eclipsed.

The intuition, which sees what is not there that should be there, has a tendency when used alone to try to force something to be there, in a vindictive manner. Intuition isolated has a justified vindication motive, which carries a sense of entitlement.

The intellect, which sees what is there that shouldn't be there, has a tendency when used alone to destroy, in a hostile manner, and carries a sense of disconnect and apathy. Intellect by itself gives a sense of justification to its hostility.

Vindictiveness and hostility seem to be similar, but the difference is, the intuition says, "I want to get my revenge by making them regret what they did," and the intellect says, "I just want them gone."

"The will" which controls how we switch perspectives in order to make the intuition and the intellect see the same thing, has a tendency to dominate and commandeer. "The will" says, "I control everything so that I will see happen what I want!" "The will" gives a sense of power as it tries to puppeteer people and things.

One thing common to all three when used isolated, is that they don't like to be opposed. When someone tells us we are wrong, the appropriate response would be, "It's impossible a hundred percent right, and very possible that I am quite a bit wrong, but I haven't figured out how I'm wrong yet, so please enlighten me." It doesn't even matter what someone is accusing us of doing. Not everyone will have something substantial to enlighten us with, but might give us just the lead we need to figure it out ourselves.

In all psychopathology, it is resistance to feeling wrong that is what pushes us to take our mind and emotions out of the equation and let our reflexes do all the work.

There is an assumption often operating that says, "If we didn't think about what we say or do, then we don't feel we consciously did anything, meaning we don't have to think about what was wrong about it, and even if someone tries to throw it in our face, it doesn't even sound familiar... because we didn't consciously do it."

There are two ways to judge, by action or by intent. If we don't do anything with conscious intention, we might assume we can't ever be guilty by intent. We often judge with both intent and action, because it is not always convenient to judge just by intent. If we want to be mad at someone, and the action doesn't actually merit being mad, we can just assume the intent. This gives us the illusion that we are in control of how we feel about things.

Since pathology comes from using any of the three systems of the psyche alone, this is not a permanent state of being, but a temporary triggered state. No one to my knowledge is free of triggers, and no one has so many that they are always triggered, we are all somewhere on that spectrum.

We also have more than one response when we are triggered. There are twenty-one different interpersonal or personal weapons, and likely we have our top three favorites. This means that when we are triggered, we likely get ourselves into any of three different problems. It doesn't mean that it is impossible to use any other weapon, the right circumstance and mood might be able to illicit the use of any of the twenty-one different weapons.

I created a survey and had ninety friends anonymously rate my use of interpersonal skills and weapons. I remember when seeing that my highest rated interpersonal weapon was persistence(which now is relentlessness), I thought, "They're just being nice, they know that's the least bad of all the weapons, and they don't want me to feel bad..." then I realized, "Hmmm... maybe it really is a problem, because I don't even really see much wrong with being persistent." I made it a focus of attention to not be persistence, and the difference was surprisingly good. The increase of contentment and composure I experienced was definitive evidence that is had been a problem. After thinking about it a lot, I figured I should switch the word I use for the weapon from persistence to relentlessness, which better describes inability to soften feeling, temper or determination when they are too harsh.

I think part of the problem, was that the different things I identified with involve perseverance, and so it would make sense that I would be inclined to overuse that tool. The root of pathology is identity. Triggers are the only way to protect an identity, because logically we can't protect it, and intuitively we won't either. Every time we are triggered, we should look into what identity we feel is at stake. We need to take advantage of our moments of clear thinking, and cross the bridges into stages of greater awareness.

The question is: "If we have the right tool in front of us, why not use it?"

There are two reasons, one, we are unfamiliar with the proper tool for the situation, or two, we feel it is taboo or not ideal because our definition for the interpersonal weapon is too inclusive and has encroached on the definition of the tool. How strong our fear of unfamiliarity and how entrenched the taboo or ideal is, will determine how pathological the response will be when that tool was the one required.

It was not my plan to include psychopathology in this book, because though it could be that each condition fits nicely behind a particular tool or be a combination, there might be overlap in conditions that appear the same but have different underlying causes, and would need to be separated and renamed. Also, there is a convention of prognosis and gravity of different psychopathology, making the distinction between personality disorders and mood disorder. My theory would show a difference in which system of the psyche is being reflexively dominating, but ultimately the process of fixing the problem would be essentially the same. Each psychopathology could come in a range of gravity, and the gravity would determine the need for hospitalization, and not the nature of the psychopathology. Also that certain weapons combined could amplify each other, leading to a more complex expression of the psychopathology, but would have the same process, addressing both weapons as we normally would.

All psychopathology is immaturity. We are not born mentally sick or get mentally sick or mentally infected. Each person has the ability to handle the complexity in life in some areas is better than others. We can all probably list our three favorite interpersonal tools and three favorite interpersonal weapons, the difference is in our awareness of our bias towards our favorite tools, and our awareness of our use of weapons.

There is a taboo in the psychology world, to ask a therapist what their cure rate is. Though the therapist knows what the person means in asking, and could give an answer, they typically dislike the question, because it is a way of measuring the psychologist on something that depends ultimately on their patients. To add to that the therapist doesn't typically see a struggle in their patient's life not being a struggle, but that a person gets better at not letting it get to them. I would say that our experience in life will always be in reference to our weaknesses, but that isn't a bad thing. Our weaknesses plague us until we decide to really face them, and then they become strengths as we change them. I think it is a matter of maturing, and not curing in psychopathology, we're naïve not broken.

Alcoholism for instance, once it is overcome, the person doesn't forget all the intricacies of the cost-benefit of alcohol once they become sober. They still know exactly what problems alcohol seemed to solve, and when faced with those problems, they cannot completely exclude it as a possible remedy. Why? For example, I personally don't drink alcohol, but I know many people who see it as a normal part of their life, and have set what they feel are appropriate bounds for its use. It is a lot easier for me, who has not experienced any benefits, but knows several disadvantages, to not see alcohol as worth it. However, similarly in my life, fully knowing both the advantages of things like soda, fast food, sleeping in, not exercising and whatever else, in the cost benefit analysis, they sometimes still win.

Every asset has associated risks, and when making a decision, while trying to optimize value, we are not picking between correct or incorrect, or right or wrong, but cost vs benefit in safe bet vs the risky bet.

Whether I can study or write better while drinking a caffeinated soda has yielded inconsistent results, but sometimes the gamble seems worth it, however drinking a soda before going to the gym has yielded consistently negative results. This is the process of maturity, and the only way to help someone mature faster, is to help them remember and process the data they have already gathered or are currently gathering. One thing that slows down this process is false information. Many cases of grave disability due to psychopathology are caused because of the burden of an overwhelming amount of counterproductive information, and limited resources of productive information.

My experience working in a psych ward as a medical student, was that not only did many people with schizophrenia have a history of methamphetamine abuse, but also that the abuse started in their earl teen years, often to cope with a history of physical or sexual abuse. I realize that the demographics of the hospitals I worked at are not representative of the world as a whole, but the trends definitely show something.

I saw that other patients with the same schizophrenia diagnosis really just had borderline or histrionic personality disorder coupled with poor coping mechanisms. They seemed to have a history of an above average difficulty developmental learning curve of unmanageable conflicts and limited accessible resources.

When we are confronted with a conflict so much more complex than our current understanding of life, it is like building a boat once you are already thrown in the water—it's a lot easier to build a boat before you get thrown in the water, especially if the water is deep. All the water has to be is an inch deeper than you can reach, and it might as well be the middle of the ocean.

For example, how many adults feel they really understand the nature and purpose of sex? I would say very few, and so when that concept is thrust on a child, it will likely be a long time before on their own they will be able to make sense of it. Just because this child will have this area of infinite dept of uncertainty in their life, doesn't mean in other aspects they will be at all delayed or affected, in fact, it is quite often the opposite. Figuring out something that seems just within our grasps seems like the best approach to getting closer to grasping something that seems out of reach. This is what gives the perplexing contrast of cognitive and emotional function which seems to be able to vary so drastically. A person can run a large business well and yet cannot handle a small criticism, meanwhile another person can talk to anyone about anything calmly and yet not be able to hold a job.

When we are incapacitated by our mind or emotion being overwhelmed, we are left to reflexes and triggers; it is not an illness that is striking us, it is a situation that demands a part of us that is not mature enough to handle it. Some things that seem relatively easy to handle for one person, another person might be completely unfamiliar with them and feel overwhelmed. A traumatic event doesn't infect us like a virus, it overwhelms into panic or hysteria depending on the discrepancy between the understanding required for a situation and the understanding we have.

It is most often difficult concepts that overwhelm us rather than actual physical obstacles. Rape or war produces post-traumatic stress disorder much more often than physical accidents, natural disasters or illness, because the emotional foundation we stand on can be shaken by ideas that can feel just as real as our perception of life. It isn't very hard to get all turned around; All it takes is one person close to us to betrays us, and everything we thought we knew is challenged, and that emotional foundation crumbles beneath us. There are many things that can shake our foundation, but the key is to have ready to use all the tools to build a foundation, and not have some of them tabooed.

"You're letting them walk all over you." "Keep your thoughts to yourself!" "Why would you do that? Are you an idiot?" "Don't be so needy." "Oh, so you're just a know-it-all…" "Do you think you own the place?" "Why didn't you do anything? You should have at least done something… anything." "Mind your own business."

The two most common difficulties are finding a balance between asserting yourself but not too much or too little, and opening up emotionally, but not too much or too little.

It's not that one tool is tabooed and another is not, likely most of them are tabooed in one way or another, and so even when we are using the right tool we second guess ourselves. Apart from all the taboos, there is also all the counterproductive ideals we grow up hearing. There is a reason we get overwhelmed, it's because so often our hands are tied, and we are in a lose-lose situation, because we assume reflexively using one system of the psyche instead of all three at least spares us from two of the three possible taboos.

The process to undo the taboos, fears and ideals limiting our ability to act, is to notice when we get triggered, and figure out why we did. The answer will always be where it is that our identity has been challenged. For example, maybe we see someone in our group not working as hard as we are, and we get angry. Really, we were working extra hard, partly so that no one could say we weren't pulling our weight, because that would be taboo. And partly, we are irritated that we feel obligated to work harder than we think we should, just to avoid shame. The anger is partly towards life which allows shame to exist, but we justify putting it on the slacker, because at least the job could get over faster if we all did our share of the work.

In the case of the slacker, it goes deeper—there is a taboo on being assertive and calling the slacker out, and there is an ideal about not complaining or snitching. There we are, feeling shame either way, and getting frustrated, and at some point, we get so triggered we just give up and let our reflexes handle it.

Though there is so much delineated in psychology with data to prove efficacy, there still are a few holes in current psychological terminology. For example, a parent that gets so triggered by their crying baby that they shake their infant until it stops crying... and ends up dying, what is that disorder? What about the person who steals money from their grandma, what diagnosis is that? Because that takes a special sort of justification to justify stealing from your grandma.

I am not proposing a new naming structure, but a foundational understanding of the possible components of the mind and emotion that can go wrong. Diagnosis is important because if someone is a risk to themselves and others, there is a large difference between psychological hospitalization and criminal imprisonment, and our diagnosis should facilitate the best outcome.

Using any of the three systems of the psyche alone in a situation will lead to vindictiveness, hostility, or domineering without really noticing it, because using only one system of the psyche isolated means we are using it like a reflex. Those can be expressed through any of the seven emotional lenses. When we are fixated in one emotional lens, we don't see why using a weapon of that lens is bad. This means that the general treatment for all psychopathologies is the same, to reframe the situation through each of the seven aspects of value, and use all three systems of the psyche in order. For each lens, what is the asset, what is the risk, what is the best way to combine those into a plan? Then after doing that for all seven aspects of value, which seems to make the biggest difference?

It is not possible to do something that doesn't have merit in at least one aspect of value, but one aspect of value is not good enough. When we make a choice, it should be positive in one aspect, and at least neutral in all other six aspects of value. Stealing money from your grandma may be in a way functional, but it is definitely not positive in any of the other aspects of value. Trying what the random thoughts or voices suggest whether they seem solid or not may be explorative, but it is not positive for any of the other aspects of value.

The first part of identifying the psychopathology is to determine which system of the psyche has a taboo, fear or ideal against it.

Tools in the intellect are typically blocked by ideals against them by the persona aspect of the ego. An ideal appears to come from within, and so the hostility is directed inward until it is vented outward.

Tools of the intuition are typically blocked by taboos against them by the shadow aspect of the ego. A taboo is something imposed from outside, and so the vindictiveness is generally directed outward, until it is vented inward.

Tools of "the will" are typically overcompensated by the ego with an ideal that over-promotes the tool, and no taboo against the corresponding weapon. Domination from the ego is usually directed toward life in general, and then vented back into one's connection with life and energy.

All psychopathology comes from feeling blindsided by an aspect of value that was not even thought to look for, that damages our sense of self by feeling taboo or not ideal, which then is over compensated for, by hyper-sensitivity and hyper-vigilance.

We are capable of entertaining three of the twenty-one pathologies at once—one in the ego, one in the persona, and one in the shadow, and they can switch between the different positions, or be traded out completely for other weapons. Psychopathology is relative to the sensitivities and complexities of one tool compared to other tools and weapons.

Whichever tool is focused on improvement, it improves faster than the others, especially when it is already used proficiently. We use aspects of value to measure things, and the more familiar with that form of measuring, the more possible measurements there can be. If you had a ruler with no marks on it, you could only conclude it was twelve inches exactly, or not. Each experience when compared and contrasted against all other ones can become a new possible measurement mark, filling in intervals of inches and quarter inches. Because of this, whichever tool is neglected becomes relatively more reactive, because instead of having exact measurements, it is either a yes or a not, a danger or safe, a do or don't.

Psychopathology could be explained as the deficit of our most immature or primitive emotional lens or system of the psyche to operate compared to the more mature other components, producing reactivity when that aspect of value is the one in question. This means, that after working on our most immature emotional lens or system to the psyche, another one would become the source of new problems as it comparably becomes the new most reactive. Improving the measurement capability of our best emotional lens increases the complexity of some components of a concept, the magnifies the shortcomings of the least familiar emotional lens, making it more reactive. This will be the model until each emotional lens and each system of the psyche is optimally mature.

Which system of the psyche the reactivity is coming from determines what general kind it will be.

Psychopathology in the shadow is rooted in the intuition, and is fundamentally vindictive, and creates an alienation from one's self, which ultimately leads to self-harm and torture of others.

Psychopathology in the ego is rooted in "the will," and is fundamentally domineering. It creates and alienation from life, which ultimately leads to psychosis.

Psychopathology in the persona is rooted in the intellect, and is fundamentally hostile, creating an alienation from others, which can ultimately lead to suicide or homicide.

The general feeling of anxiety is the intellect trying to take rightful control of the situation. The general feeling of depression is the intuition trying to take rightful control of the situation.

I do not have a complete delineation of the complications of reactivity in each of the twenty-one different interpersonal tools, but they could be assumed from the general convention previously provided. There are however some conditions in the current diagnostic criteria of psychology where this convention elicits some new understanding and approaches for treatment. I will include only a select few conditions that are explained very well with this approach.

These are tentative conceptualizations of certain thought processes and their corresponding psychopathologies that precipitate. Just like the progression of type 2 diabetes, where the intake of sugar creates a change in the presence of hormones, which then changes tissues, which in turn changes production of hormones, the same is true of psychopathologies. It becomes a chemical imbalance, but the inciting factor was a thought process, and so medications can help us overcome the chemical imbalance while we change the thought process that started it.

I hesitate to even add this part, because I don't want people throwing around diagnosis or labeling themselves with disorders, but I still feel this could be more helpful than hurtful. It is at the back of the book for a reason, so that once you gotten to this point in the book, the idea will more likely be received in the right context.

That context is: We all have sources of stress, it will come through what interpersonal weapons we have overly strong taboos for. That stress will manifest in any of twenty-one different ways, which will be the interpersonal weapons you think are least bad. Depending on our coping mechanisms and how strong or weak the taboos are, will determine how much that stress will effect our ability to function. Just because we are functioning better than average, or even better than most, doesn't mean that the stress isn't holding us back from doing a lot more, and enjoying it better.

The weakest link in a chain is where it will break. That isn't to say that a chain isn't strong, the strongest chain in the world still has one link where if measured would be the weakest, and if it were to break, it would be where the break would occur. That list that you made back at the beginning of the book, take the three interpersonal weapons you rated as least bad, and see which diagnosis have those weapons involved. This does not mean you clinically have this disorder, it means that when the pressure of a situation gets strong enough, that is the way the stress will manifest. A clinical diagnosis means that someone is affecting our ability to function so much that it merits clinical attention. For example, someone could have rated complaining as the least bad interpersonal weapon and still be very functional even when a situation is very difficult, but when stress does come, it will come in the form of Chronic Depression.

The weakest link in the chain works well to explain why simply labeling and medicating someone doesn't work very well. The symptoms we feel when we are stressed are indicators of which link is the weakest. We then can strengthen it, and then endure more stress than before, but that doesn't mean we can endure any stress. A subsequent stressor bigger than what we could handle before will show us what our new weakest link is.

It's not a coincidence that when I first outlined the interpersonal tools, that I thought relentlessness was the least bad, and that I have stayed up countless nights working on this book in a manic sort of state. It's debatable how functional that is, but why I bring this up, was as soon as I realized it was a problem, I strengthened that link in my chain, and the next big stressor after that manifested in a very different way. Apparently the next least bad interpersonal weapon for me was provoking pity, because I did something very borderline. I don't have all the twenty-one possible ways stress can manifest outlined, and so it's hard to say which it changed to after I realized provoking pity was the weakest chain. I am not holding on to how my stress has manifested as something that defines me, but rather stepping stones for having an overall stronger chain that can withstand the strain of life sufficient enough to carry it well.

Panic disorder:
Panic comes from reactivity(hypersensitivity) in the anger emotional lens, in the intellect system of the psyche. Specifically, there is a taboo placed on the tool honesty because it seems to come across as aggressive which is looked at as negative, and a taboo on its corresponding weapon, deceit. There is anxiety when we try to find some way around what seems like a lose-lose situation, where either we will offend someone by being honest, or feel guilty for lying.

Anger is an important emotional lens for confidence, because its aspect of value is resolve or stability. The general tool of anger is assertiveness, and because it has been blocked from use because of taboos and ideals against it, it has not been developed as much as other tools and is relatively primitive in comparison. The fundamental characteristic of an instance of psychological immaturity is splitting. In the case of Panic disorder, what is being split is conditions of acceptable assertiveness, creating reactivity in the circumstance when the question whether to assert one's self is presented.

These conditions of assertiveness, lead to a general tendency to avoid asserting one's self, or asserting too much. Asserting too much leads to a stronger taboo against anger, and anxiety of future instances of over-assertion.

The less we assert ourselves, the less we will see ways to do it successfully, which means the more trapped we will feel because we will see less viable options for assertiveness.

Trapped on a road with seemingly no exits, producing anxiety of what opportunities are being passed up, is how we feel. Because of this, there is a tendency to impulsively veer off the road where there is no logical exit to feel anything but being trapped. This typically produces a consequent regret of that choice, because likely we find there was nothing in the random spot we veered off, partly because the choice to veer off was when the regret of missed opportunities was maximal, not when we actually saw an opportunity. Those instances of self-assertion seem anticlimactic because of the insecurity of the consequences of breaking the taboo make it harder to explore the possibilities of asserting. We then feel more trapped because not only are we restricted by the taboo against self-assertion, but also not finding much worth blazing a new trail for, and can we become apathetic towards the idea. Alone on the highway of life is how we are prone to feel.

Hostility in the case of panic disorder is directed inward at one's right to assert themselves, and confidence is destroyed. When confidence is critically low, whatever the next possibility to assert ourselves, we will likely impulsively do, by destroying whatever or whoever is or might oppose us.

The hyper-sensitivity and hyper-vigilance is toward the consequence of self-assertion. Treatment would start by making a journal of times you asserted yourself and it went okay. It also might help to tell close friends that you would like to enlist their help finding the boundaries and balance of asserting yourself. We can let others know we want to be more honest, open and assertive, and would like them to tell us if we are asserting ourselves too much in something—that way we don't have to do so much guessing about it. Doing this we will find that boundaries we thought were there, aren't really there. That people, especially friends, want us to feel comfortable speaking our mind.

We probably don't realize that not speaking our mind can show that we don't trust the person we are talking to, because likely we feel we are not speaking our mind because we don't trust ourselves. Creating an agreement in a friendship that both should feel comfortable speaking their mind, and comfortable telling the other person when they are being too pushy, is a very healthy element to a relationship.

If we unbiasedly increase value and apply logic where we see it, most of what we see will involve ourselves, and that's okay. Although it is easier to notice something good in someone else and want to add to it, or something bad we want to change, only being able to change ourselves, it is often better to start there. It is sort of like on the plane when the stewardess says that in an emergency to put the air mask on yourself first before helping someone else. This is not only because you can't help someone else if you pass out, but also because you can put a mask on yourself faster than you can someone else.

This also has to do with the fact that it is a lot easier to help someone else, after you have already practiced the change in yourself. I made a rule for myself, that when I see something in someone else I would like to help them change, I have to find something parallel or similar in my own life and change that first. In order to help a friend quit smoking, though it was usually only one can of soda a day, I quit drinking my favorite flavor soda. I thought it would be no big deal, but quitting the soda apparently had a surprising emotional component I wasn't expecting. It gave me insight to my friend's struggle with tobacco.

It isn't always an investment or change in ourselves that has to come first, our intuition will spontaneously suggest things we can do to help or support others, and that's fine. Since those impulses to invest are spontaneous, that means that more ideas of where to invest will spontaneously be directed towards ourselves just because we are around ourselves most, and that's okay.

Psychoanalyst Karen Horney wrote in New Ways in Psychoanalysis, "First, anxiety appeared when she wished something for herself which she could not justify on the grounds of needing it for education, health, and the like; second, she was subject to frequent attacks of fatigue which covered up an impotent rage…" Rage is a weapon of the anger emotional lens, but of the intuition instead of the intellect. This is why the anger lens keeps feeling like the right aspect of value, and why the intuitive anger tool enthusiasm is used until it turns to rage.

We don't have to avoid people in order to hoard our own energies, and we also don't have to be a slave to make other people happy. It is not our job to make others happy, and it isn't practical to live in such a way that we are always ecstatic about life. It is our job to look for value, and add to it where we see best. Yes, there are some things we do that drain our energy, but strictly controlling energy using enthusiasm isn't the answer. At a certain point prudence becomes totalitarian asceticism, when that happens, we are doing more harm than help.

Treatment would greatly be helped by making a very detailed list of goals and aspirations and arranging them in order of priority. We often find ourselves trying to maintain a perfect score at one goal, at the expense of another goal of higher priority, because we feel less trapped or guilty for missing other opportunities if we have one thing that is perfect. Pleasing people cannot be the number one priority, that goal has to be much more specific—in which ways and at what costs we please people must be delineated. Most often our decisions are between a safe gamble and a risky gamble, not between good or bad, or smart or stupid. If we merely have the goal to please people, we would be tempted to always go with the safe gamble for accomplishing it. Anxiety builds against this risk aversion, which means that when a risk is presented, the accompanying anxiety is feared, making the risk even harder to weigh out with the distracting anxiety. This process soon produces aversion to decision in general.

An example in my own life, in racing motocross, one day, a portion of the track was accidently flooded, and had more than two feet of mud. There was no way of getting through that section without getting muddy. I found my best hope, was to turn the corner as wide as possible and come at the muddy section as straight and as fast as possible. There was no use dreading that section of the track every lap, and no use complaining that the mud made my whole bike slippery. If we are cleaning our room, it is very possible to have it be spotless, and completely organized, life is not like our room, and that's okay, it's fine to get a little muddy sometimes. The important thing is to remember our priorities, and not panic when circumstances make it so hard that only the top one of two priorities are possible. We can either avoid that section of track by quitting the race, or get muddy and gain experience so the next time we go through it we are better.

For us keeping every commitment we make is a priority, but keeping every commitment and resenting the people we made commitments to is not a good trade-off. I would say a good friend is someone that keeps about eighty percent of their commitments to me. If a friend is weighing out a decision, I don't want them factoring in me possibly being mad, I hope they know I will be understanding. We have to trust that the investments we have made in the past are still worth something, friendship is not like the stock market that could crash overnight. Even in extreme circumstances when friendship seems to come apart instantly, it's hard to not still think or care about the other person. And so, if even the most extreme circumstances can't sever a friendship completely, we shouldn't assume something little would.

A big part of what drives the priority to please people is the identity of being agreeable and selfless. It is nice when people recognize that we are selfless enough to want to make them happy, but we shouldn't let recognition be the priority. Putting ourself in the other person's perspective helps. Would you want your friend to have a mental break down because they are scared to tell you that they are too stressed to be able to make the lunch appointment they had promised? This is why reactivity in the intellect causes alienation from others, because we entertain assumptions about what they would do or feel that are completely unrelatable.

I have a really good friend that often calls me on his way to work or when running errands, and I actually feel glad to know that even mid-sentence, that if he has to go, he just says, "one sec," then hangs up. It is even more confirming of the trust he has in our friendship, that after saying "one sec," he knows that even if he doesn't have time to call back that day or even the next, that I'm not at all bothered by it.

Connection is a synergy, which means life should be easier with a friend not harder. Assuming others have strict expectations of us can make friendship seem like a burden sometimes. We often give our friends the benefit of the doubt and hold the assumption that they don't intend to let us down or hurt us, we should assume they are giving us the same benefit of the doubt.

Obsessive Compulsive disorder:

Obsessive compulsive disorder comes from reactivity in the intuition system of the psyche through the anger lens, corresponding to the tool enthusiasm, and the weapon rage.

A key part of both Enthusiasm and rage is anticipation, because the time we spend preparing for something sensitizes us. When we aren't anticipating anything, it can pass us by completely unnoticed. When we are anticipating something, we can think we see it everywhere. Similar to how we are more prone to being more aggressive than we should when we feel we are trapped, depending on what we feel trapped by, and what we think would be the best place to focus our aggression, will determine how it goes. The "release" associated with OCD, is from the strain of the anticipation, because the idea is, "if I do ____ I won't have to anticipate it till it's done, or anticipate the repercussions of nothing having done it." If we are not aware of what we are anticipating or why, it can consume us.

Obsessive compulsive disorder is a hyper-sensitivity centered mostly on attacks on one's self-esteem, through either self-criticism or criticism from others. Because the anger lens is responsible for the question of assertiveness, when there is a problem that we could fix with being assertive, but someone won't let us, we have to find a way to work around them. Chaos compels assertion, and because we are trying to avoid being assertive in order to not damage a relationship, then we try to control chaos by bringing order to it. When someone blames us for something that is not our fault, or mostly not our fault, if experience has show us that we can't just defend ourselves, we have to be above reproach—we have to make sure no accidents are caused by us.

If we want to influence someone, but they get irritated easily, we have to influence them indirectly, by paving the way for them so that the easiest road to take is the one we have laid out. When we have time to prepare or craft a situation things usually work flawlessly, but when we get rushed, or when people bring chaos into the situation it makes it very difficult.

People seem to have a very low tolerance for us to be assertive, but there is no limit to how much we can assert ourselves on inanimate objects, in fact, we are usually praised for it; it is indirect-assertion. This assertion on things instead of people also seems to have the added benefit of eliminating the possible criticism by doing things to perfection.

In reality assertion can be direct or indirect depending on the situation, but for us who have had countless bad experiences with confrontation when we are assertive try to exclusively be indirectly assertive, but asserting ourselves on everything around ourselves or other people instead of assertive with the other person. There is a certain amount of energy or enthusiasm that builds in order to be assertive, and when that energy should be directed towards something or someone that we know will become confrontational, we channel it into something inanimate, or disguise our assertiveness behind motives of cleanliness or order.

Anger's aspect of value is resolve or stability, and its fundamental action is to hold, and so in order to hold onto the permanence of respect of ourselves, we feel, we have to change the environment to fit us, so that we don't let the environment be the means of self-criticism and thereby the means of controlling us. Strength is rooted in the anger lens, and obsessive compulsiveness is a way to gain strength over self-criticism and criticism from others.

Treatment would be similar to that of the panic disorder, namely, that speaking our mind is important, specifically our feelings. Thinking that our friends or even people in general expect perfection in order to appreciate us is not putting a lot of confidence in our friends or humanity. Yes, not everyone wants to hear our opinion, there is probably a specific person we want to speak our mind to and haven't, and every time we think about it we do something OCD to distract ourselves. We have to consider whether it is worth it, and if it is, just talk straight to that person, and if it isn't, remember that you are making a conscious decision not to, not because you are scared to be assertive, but that the pros don't outweigh the cons.

Each action we do should have some sort of expectation from it, preferably the more valuable and logically the better. If we have already washed our hands once, what do we hope happens when we wash them again? If we just want to be distracted from the person we can't be assertive with, there are a lot of better distractions than washing your hands again.

It would also be good to learn to do something new, and writing about the experience, specifically the things about the journey that were enjoyed not the outcome. Write about what things along that journey we incidentally find by mistake fumbling our way through. It would help to have a friend join in the process, but isn't absolutely necessary. Since what reinforces the tendency of OCD is being results oriented, look for things to complement in others and yourself that aren't results oriented, and actually compliment them.

Mania:

Mania is reactivity in the will-power system of the psyche through the anger lens, which tool is perseverance, and weapon is relentlessness. Mania happens when there is an ideal promoting perseverance, and no taboo on the weapon of relentlessness. This creates a feedback cycle of increasing input of energy and determination directed both inward and outward until the all energy and determination is depleted and there is a crash.

Being a psychopathology in the will-power, that in this case it means that the domineering tendency from the ego is directed toward life in general, and one's towards one's own life and energy.

Treatment would follow the general course of the other two anger lens psychopathologies, Panic and OCD, where the general concept is to not assume that worthiness for connection is results oriented. Specifically in the case of mania, the task is to identify the obstacle that we feel requires relentlessness to push past. Then assess whether the obstacle principally feels like something that you are trying to prove, or principally that you want to do. It is not necessary nor possible to assess exactly how much our motives are to prove, but if it feels like close or more than fifty percent, it would probably be wise to re-evaluate whether we should push so hard to make it happen.

A problem with mania is that the energy gets directed in many different directions, not all of which are important— proving we can do something leads us to push forward ideas we don't really care about. We should make a list of priorities, and invest the bulk of our energy in top priorities. When a new idea comes, we should compare and contrast it against the list.

Chronic Depression:

Chronic Depression is reactivity in the intuition system of the psyche, specifically of the disgust lens, where there is a taboo on appreciating, and no taboo on the weapon complaining.

After being blindsided by something degrading, a hypervigilance and hypersensitivity occurs in the momentum we have towards overcoming obstacles.

What blindsides us in chronic depression is often big, and if we overcame it, the knowledge and character strength gained are big assets. In this case because we have done great things, our standards of excellence for ourselves exceeds our assessment of our ability. We have a high standard for ourselves of what is worth appreciating. We don't do it on purpose, but complaining does make an accomplishment in hindsight feel greater. Complaining however also makes the obstacle in the present seem more daunting.

Resulting battle scares seem to be solid evidence that what we did was hard enough to appreciate the work we put in to overcome it.

In chronic depression there is a tendency to create small obstacles as a way to gain momentum by overcoming them in preparation for an eminent larger obstacle.

Being part of the intuition, chronic depression isn't conscious, and so when talked about logically it doesn't make sense and sounds insensitive. Chronic depression should be primarily communicated non-verbally using hugs. This may seem odd, but how long it takes someone to relax in a hug shows how they are doing, and in chronic depression it is the most accurate way to know how someone is.

In chronic depression there is some self-defeating behavior, because each failed attempt proves the difficulty of the obstacle, so that when it is overcome, there is more reason to appreciate it.

Criticism is the main obstacle that we try to avoid, because what blindsided us, has been used against us to shame us instead of be a symbol of what we have overcome. This creates a sensitivity to others minimizing our problems and shaming us; this pressures us to figure out how to explain the degrading event more clearly, or emotionally charge it so others perceive it for what it is. There is a tendency to practice defending against this criticism by criticizing ourselves.

Self-criticism in a way seems motivating, because it gives us something to prove, and when we lack the energy, the possible shame that will come if we give up pushes us to keep going.

There is an apprehension to move beyond the degradation incident, because as it is forgotten, the grandeur of it is minimized, and when it is minimized, all the behavior to promote its grandeur would then seem ridiculous.

The weapon of complaining reinforces the cycle. The tool of appreciation puts the focus on the positive. Like all weapons of the intuition, there is a fundamental vindictive nature, which is most often pointed inwards. In chronic depression there is a low tolerance for hostility, because in chronic depression the majority of the negative energy is directed inward, which means we are already carrying a heavy load, and we are not doing anything to other people so any aggression towards us seems totally unwarranted. We don't realize that hurting ourselves hurts other people, and so when people try to get involved it usually just comes across as hostile.

Like all pathology in the shadow, the question should be asked, "what am I trying to force to be there that I think isn't there?"

The vindictive nature of the shadow holds on to the self-destructive cycle, because at some point it hopes to make the perpetrator of the degradation regret what they did. They feel that if they let go, that would be letting them escape or even condoning the terrible action.

The treatment would be to start a gratitude journal. Also pick a person and write them a letter telling them everything you appreciate about them. Pick a new person every week or month. Only allow yourself a certain amount of time to think about the past, like no more than thirty minutes a day. Thoughts can be written down to be considered once a week, and what is thought must be written down, and have a conclusion that motivates specific action. Try to make the conclusions concise, and then every once in a while, combine all previous conclusions into one concise life philosophe.

Manic depression:

Manic depression is a psychopathology in "the will" system of the psyche, specifically of the disgust lens. It is an ideal on the tool hope, and an ideal in weapon skepticism.

Manic depression could be conceptualized as an arm wrestle with one's self. We feel if we prove hope can avail, then we are allowed to have hope in life and be content. However, there is also an ideal for skepticism, which leads to feeling that if we are able to be as realistic as possible and scrutinize everything, we are allowed to feel safe and prepared. This irony puts maximal energy forward while at the same time maximal resistance against forward movement, creating an unbearable strain. We feel like we are always working hard, but surprised to find after several hours go by sometimes we have done a ridiculous amount of work, while other times we have done nothing. The energy commitment is usually there, but this does not mean we can depend on ourselves to actually get anything done.

Since not all the hope, nor all the skepticism in manic depression is misguided, we do actually figure out quite a bit, and at times do blaze an impressive trail of success until we trip up and lose our momentum. Once our momentum is gone, we have a terrible time building it back up against the friction of our own and other people's skepticism.

Criticism from others is both appreciated and feared. We always think we can take it, and one thing at a time we can, but the pace normal criticism comes anyway, and the criticism we invite builds up, and once we lose our footing, we buckle under the weight of it. We feel we have to process all of it and find out of the criticism what helps us transcend obstacles, but some things take more time and energy to process and we get backlogged. Not only do we process all criticism we can, but everything people do and say we analyze for variables in the equation of life.

There is a paradox in this situation about whether connection with others is worth it, because other people add too many variables to scrutinize, and so anything but small groups at the most, with people we trust, is the energy required to scrutinize everything bearable. People are both a source of what needs to be scrutinized, but also a source of hope, and so we are torn between being with people and being alone.

The overabundance of hope makes us likeable, and so though we likely don't initiate social gatherings, we are often invited, but prefer the small ones. There is a little tension in our friendships, because most others don't know what to do with that much hope and skepticism combined—it makes them nervous, because situations can seem to change rapidly. Someone may feel like everything in a situation is normal, and our mind in a manic depressive state has already been a hundred places and come to some radical conclusion. This tendency to make radical conclusions is hard to debunk, because sometimes we are right, and other times there is no way of disproving it.

Treatment would be to avoid the tendency to build assumptions without testing them, and to not make assumptions about people when we can just ask them personally. We need to bring people into our world. Asking sincere questions that help us get to know someone does several things; it helps us make less assumptions, it slows our thinking down so that we don't get too far separated from others in the same room, and it helps us see less danger, because having a sincere conversation usually promotes friendship, and the more friends we have, the easier to manage a difficult situation. When we gain a friend we also lose a possible enemy.

Post Traumatic Stress Disorder:

Post traumatic stress disorder is reactivity in the intellect, specifically in the disgust lens, where there is a taboo on humor, and no taboo against dogmatization. Humor is room we give for how we see the big picture of life to change, and the ability to consider all possible options of integration of new ideas. Humor is what balances out the rigidity of seriousness. Humor still has a productive aim, it just does it in a playful manner.

Growing up, our concept of life didn't often change, and the big picture never seems drastically wrong-it seemed rich with nostalgia. Our first assumption of life is likely that it is good, or at least not malevolent. At some point, when we first see something that doesn't fit anywhere in our concept of the world, a lot of things have to move to make room for it. Often this is our first exposure to malevolence, whether it was someone else who did something unbelievably wrong, or us who did something we never knew we were capable of. We then feel there is clearly nowhere in our concept of life for this new horrible thing, and we are torn between completely starting a new darker picture of life to fit this new very real feeling malevolent thing, or try to keep the old picture and ignore the new event.

It is scary to get rid of our old big picture of life, because there are a lot of things we liked about it—it becomes difficult to imagine nostalgia and fantastical aspirations from the old picture of life still having a place in the new darker picture. We try to keep both, and our context for experience flickers back and forth between the two big pictures. This creates two fears, the fear of the malevolence recurring, and the fear of how drastically perspective shifts when the old and new pictures switch. It is scary to think how drastically the dark picture might change our response to normal life.

The latter fear, of what happens when the map switches, creates a distrust of self, which leads to self-isolation as a precaution to others, and decreases how relatable others appear. This means reaching out to find a solution seems unnatural, not to mention even if the other person has experienced a trauma, they likely try not to talk about it.

There is also a hypervigilance and hypersensitivity toward betrayal, creating a splitting, where instead of noticing a slight increase in risk, the psyche goes into full alarm mode. Our nerves put others around them on edge, which change in others is noticed, and full out war is prepared for.

Since it is a pathology of the intellect, it is fundamental nature is hostile towards others, which is often repressed because of the feeling of alienation from others arounds us.

The intellect is the engineering function, it sees risks to subtract, and there seems nothing humorous about considering risks, but there has to be, because we don't have a perfect understanding of risks, and meanings and motives we attribute to things are often bias and incomplete.

Each asset in life has very specific risks associated with it, and it is a matter of identifying each, and then preparing against or accepting the associated risks. What happens in a traumatic situation, is that there is one asset, "life," and a myriad of risks, which means, that anytime "life" is thought about or seems threatened in any way, all the risks we have associated with it come to mind as well.

If the assets in life are clearly separated, and the appropriate risks attached to each, when one specific asset is thought of, only the associated risks will come with it, and it will be manageable.

When we look at life being the only asset, specifically life as it is, or what we are working towards, and when we look at the risk as change and pain, all our defenses will be lumped together and react at the same time anything starts to change. Also, we will be hypervigilant of possible change or pain, so that we can't enjoy life when there is no change or pain. This is one of the reasons why having a dog after trauma can help, because dogs are very vigilant, even while sleeping a suspicious noise will wake them up. This allows us to put some of the burden of vigilance on them, while we do the work of defining the actual assets and risks at play.

Post trauma, the assets are vague and the risks are very specific, and so the intellect is emphasized, which leads us to look only for what can be subtracted from the situation. The way our mind is set up to approach life, is to assess what assets are at play, and what we could add to the situation, then what risks are at play, and how we can subtract them. Lastly, because what we intuitively think of to add is a whole idea, and what we intellectually think of to subtract is a whole idea, they both have to be assessed, and the best from each can be blended into an optimum plan.

The treatment for Post Traumatic stress disorder would start with defining the assets at play. If life feels at risk, define what life is. Allow for more space for ideas and emotions, it's okay to stretch the canvas we are painting life on, there is a lot to fit in. When you feel triggered, reframe the situation in reference to all seven aspects of value; we can't define life in one dimension, and we can't see it through one or even just two emotional lenses, it won't make any sense. Also avoid dogmatically labeling things, one person is not the hero or the life of a party, we can manage a higher resolution of what is actually going on than that. There are things worth repeating, and things not, identity doesn't play into life, even though it sometimes feels like it should.

The traumatic experience should be drawn or written out, and connected to real life. If there is one picture that contains everything, then there is no switching.

Write down a life statement. Make the first line your core belief, and build off of it. When life seems to crash, look back over that life statement and find where there were exceptions to the rule, and redefine them. The reason a trauma sticks out so much in our mind, is because it is the reference file for all the assumptions about life that came from it. Once we identity those assumptions, and then test them, that experience will be our new reference file for our current assumptions about life.

Write out the whole incident of the trauma, and then with different colors highlight or write notes in the side to identity which principles each part belongs to. Make a list of those principles and define them. Then take all those principles and make a belief that connects them all. Ones those principles and beliefs have been tested and what was useful kept, and what wasn't thrown out, we can move on. When those memories are asked about, they will feel like old news, we already gleaned everything that was worth keeping and debunked the rest.

Diagraming or writing out the event and how it ties into normal life, reframing the situation into each of the seven aspects of value, will show how someone seeing a situation through only one or two lenses, could do something very terrible. Also, looking at what interpersonal weapons were used, and which tools should have been used instead helps to show that the situation in the future could be approached better. Also, knowing that we all use interpersonal weapons at times, and because we have spent so much time justifying them, that the different ones that other people use seem worse.

Substance abuse:

Substance abuse is reactivity in "the will" system of the psyche, in the contempt lens. There is ideal for the tool teamwork, and no taboo on leeching. There is a "Whatever gets the job done" and "what's mine is yours and what's yours is mine" mentality. Alcoholism goes under this psychopathology, because though harm will come from the excessive alcohol consumption on the body, it helps to function better in the moment, helps to not get irritated with other people, and helps to speak your mind. The consequences don't seem like a bad thing, because it is looked at as taking one for the team. "The team needs me now, I am willing to pay later for it."

Leeching can be in the form of emotional support or financial resources. A substance like alcohol or a stimulant is leeching from one's self. Similarly leeching from a friend or family member feel like merely leeching from ourself, because we are very willing to give resources or emotional support back more than we take.

Treatment is in not trying to balance the scale of what we give and what we take, it is about figuring out what the purpose of the teams we are on, and what the cost is. A timeline of what positive things the team has done and negative things can be made, and a plan to increase the positives and decrease the negative. Wanting to do kind or productive things is not the same as doing them, sitting around drinking and talking about doing something doesn't count as doing it.

Other people are not responsible for our happiness or luxury. The difference between needs and wants should be defined, and constantly re-evaluated. Each thing we want to ask or do, we can consider which need or want it specifically would fulfil, how we think it would fulfil it, and what the cost would be. We shouldn't feel like a burden when we ask something from someone, but we should do our part first by figuring out what we are actually asking for first.

Anti-social or Conduct disorder:

Anti-social or conduct disorder are reactivity in the contempt lens, in the intellect system of the psyche where the tool is leadership and the weapon is manipulation. Often it seems aggressiveness typically gets the job done. Anti-social doesn't mean that you are not a fan of being social, it means being against society, by having reduced regard for social boundaries or less care for what does harm to others.

The splitting is in this case is in whether or not someone is making the situation easier or harder. If the conclusion is that it is harder, whatever gets them out of the equation fastest seems like the best choice.

The decision to end a relationship, romantic or business oriented is a question of whether it has worth or doesn't, and so contempt is often the lens it is seen through, and this is why those situations among others if there is reactivity in the contempt lens can result in antisocial behavior. When anti-social behavior comes out, we are not factoring in the consequences the other person, and anything can be carelessly thrown out. For example, during a break-up someone's things are thrown out an apartment window with no thought to who it might fall on and what that would do. Or starting a fist fight without any care for possible legal, physical or emotional consequences.

Treatment would start by defining your goals. It is impossible to know how much someone or something is helping towards your goals if they are vague. If we don't give it thought, our goals will be vague, for example, the goal of a relationship might only be to not feel alone. A business goal might merely be to make money, which would mean at any cost. A friendship goal could be to be for us to feel appreciated, which would make us hard for someone else to appreciate because we are using them. If we have many clearly defined goals outlined, likely every person will at least seem helpful with one of them, even if that goal is to learn patience.

Borderline personality disorder:

Borderline personality disorder is reactivity in the intuition system of the psyche, specifically in the fear lens. There is a taboo on the tool patience, because of an assumption that someone always put first what has the most worth, in order words that the number one priority is always the focus. There is also no taboo on the weapon of provoking pity. In this situation, lack of attention given feels like an attack on self-worth.

In borderline there is a fear of loss of attachment. When fear is the focus, intuitively we are very observant of others, and make very intricate concepts of others, weighing their good and bad. Though we don't use this concept to determine the worth of others, we do that to ourselves. To combat the self-criticism, we split our concept of ourselves, separating our good and our bad, making an overly good concept, and overly bad concept. Like when someone doesn't like it if the food on their plate touches.

If intuitive fear is reactive, there is a tendency to do self-harm in our emotional lows to test whether people will still love us at our worst, so we can be sure that being at our best is definitely worth attention. Since at our best we are extremely caring with a palpable emotional investment, we often get a lot of attention, but when that attention settles, we fear that if others see our bad side, they will reject us. And so we are tempted to test whether people will reject us at our worst.

When can put ourselves at our worst we've noticed that it puts others at their best by creating a situation where in a crisis, they can step up to be a hero. In a crisis situation it seems people are forced to pay attention, or forced to show that they care if they do.

It makes it really hard to form an intricate concept of someone if they hide their thoughts and feelings, and putting ourself into a crises outweighs the fear someone has of being open and vulnerable over the fear they have for our life in peril.

If we are fixated on intuitive fear, then we are likely to assume other people do to, and we have overcome fear, and are willing to put ourself or our emotions in danger, to give others the opportunity to step up and be heroic—because we are facilitating the other person stepping up, this means that even when someone is helping us, we feel like we are teaching them.

Treatment would start by recognizing the times when we feel like we have to teach someone, and writing out how we think that would go, and then eliminate all the drastic measures, along with anything besides just supporting and encouraging the other person. Also, we should abandon the idea that we are the teacher, because odds are what we know is not much better, or in some ways actually worse, and because of our own perceptional bias, we wouldn't know that our idea isn't good. If we really think our idea is good, then write it out in a format others would want to read. If we can't put our idea in a way others are interested in, it's useless trying to force it on them.

Teaching someone is difficult because we all learn things in different orders and measure success in different ways. For example, the fear emotional lens has a reflexive mitigation to barricade, meanwhile someone else who principally uses the surprise lens is trying to explore, and so doesn't want a big bulky barricade to carry around or hide inside. There is no use suggesting what we have found to be a good barricade to someone else who doesn't see value in barricades. That would be like telling someone who is looking for a truck what your favorite car or van is.

234 | Conflict and Connection

We shouldn't make ourselves a martyr to teach others how to love, all we can do is just love. When talking with someone, try to figure out what they are trying to learn, and support them in that. The best way to support someone in what they are doing is just be genuinely interested in them. Also, maybe more importantly, find something you want to learn from them. Dr. Jordan Peterson in his book, <u>12 Rules for Life</u>, rule 9 is: "Assume that the person you are listening to might know something you don't," which is an important thing to remember when the urge to assume the teaching role appears in a situation. If we enter each conversation with the intent to learn something from someone else, we will find we learn something ourselves and inadvertently become a teacher by example.

Intake Restriction Disorder:
 Intake restriction disorder is reactivity in the intuition system of the psyche, specifically in the surprise lens. There is no taboo against intolerance when directed towards ourself because doing that seems to us like self-control, and we have an ideal towards not tolerating ourself doing anything we think we shouldn't do. The problem is if the pivotal aspect of value is perspective, then intolerance is the opposite of what should be used; self-control is only productive if we already have the right perspective. Where resolve is the aspect of value, then the interpersonal tools enthusiasm, perseverance or honesty should be the right tool, not when we don't know yet what to be enthusiastic about yet.
 Self-control is a matter of enthusiasm, perseverance and honesty in order—these three are all a completely different emotional lens than surprise. Intolerance tries to be all three at the same time. The anger lens is avoided because there is often a taboo on anger, which is where actual self-control comes from.
 Specifically in food intake restriction disorder, the reason that the surprise emotion is the pivotal one in the case of food, is because diet is not an exact science, and it is a long adventure to figure out what is optimal to eat and how much to eat. There is also so much misinformation in circulation, that when we are open-minded to all the things people say not to eat, then soon everything becomes taboo to eat. Diet is a common form of intake restriction.
 Because money and time are factors in what food we have time to buy or make, sometimes we have to settle for something sub-optimal. For example, considering the question, "would it be better to go without food all day, or eat a donut?" If

we have had good food intake for a while, it is fine to go a day without food without any negative effects on our body, but not more than a day. Our brain needs sugar to function, the rest of our body can metabolize fat for energy, but not our brain, and so going without food often will cause a strain on our brain.

The whole purpose of the surprise lens is to explore what we don't know. We can't know what we will find before we find it. We can't be intolerant about what we find. Once we find something, the we can exercise self-control.

We can't see exactly what is happening in our body, from the outside all we know is when our weight fluctuates or energy fluctuates, but those can be for for several different reasons, and we can't be intolerant about it. We also can't use a physical factor like our weight to measure our internal matter like self-control. When we choose not to eat something or choose to exercise, it should not be shame motivated, it shouldn't have anything to do with identity.

The treatment would be to write down all your aspirations, and then write how food or whatever else is being restricted, has to do with those aspirations. Attribute a pivotal aspect of value to each of those connection to food, but also assess with each lens. A good decision will be at least positive in one, and neutral in the other six. If there are any aspirations that don't meet this standard then decide how that aspiration must be modified to not be in relation to food.

In the category of things being restricted, the rationale behind avoiding them should be rated by confidence level. Make a list, and then start testing them and seeing how accurate your rating system is. Avoiding conformation bias will be difficult, but really get into the science of it and figure it out. Draw up a map from cause to effect, and consult specialists to help fill in the gaps. Also, make sure that any role model you have is someone you can actually talk to, so that you can see their whole life picture, otherwise it would be difficult to see the side effects of that lifestyle.

Burn Out:

Burn out is reactivity in the will, specifically the fear lens, which corresponds with the interpersonal weapon competitiveness. Competition is good, but we can't be competing with everyone in everything at all times forever, we can do it for a little bit, and then we will get burn out. The fear emotional lens has an unconscious reflex to mitigate by barricading. The means that we look as success as a barricade that we build up around us to protect us. If our previous successes don't precede us, and we don't know how to measure success in a situation, or we don't think success is possible, we are tempted to just give up.

Burn out is not depression or anxiety. Maybe it just feels like being sick to our stomach or that a situation seems flavorless. A more concise explanation will be in the next book. This was a late addition to this book, but a recent survey showed that it was the most common interpersonal tool people considered least bad, and so I felt obligated to include it even if I don't have it delineated very well.

Treatment could probably start with allowing yourself to be loved, in other words being vulnerable and present. You have to be able to see yourself not in reference to your success. You have to offer just your love, not dressed up in success. The 8-second hug could be very helpful. It may be hard on a daily basis to find a friend to give an 8-second hug to, but at least a few times a week should be manageable. If you don't have a friend, go visit a grandparent, or adopt a grandparent. Visiting or adopting a grandparent has the added benefit that they have enough experience in life to really measure success, and almost any grandparent knows that we are enough as we are. That doesn't mean we shouldn't be motivated to improve, but feeling we are a failure isn't the way to motivate ourselves. Have someone teach you something they like to do for fun, woodworking, knitting, checkers, etc. If you are doing it and feel you are wasting your time, write down the reasons why you think it is a waste of time, and compare and contrast it to what you think you should be doing. Making a list of long term goals and what you hope comes from each would be helpful.

The problem with competing is that more often a game is presented to us or we are pushed into it rather than choosing it ourselves. This means that the payout from winning likely won't sustain or motivate us. If the payout is to set a precedence, that precedence can be broken in an instant. If our payout is the action itself, then it can't be broken or taken from us.

Research Possibilities

There is a testable link between which of the seven emotional lenses we are perceiving life through and posture, senses, and language. This link often has a lot to do with earliest memories which show a pattern of three out of the seven emotional lenses being use for almost everything. This could be confirmed by testing recall or assessment of similar experience, using functional MRI or testing behavior choices.

1) The direct correlation between emotion and what is being perceived could be tested using functional MRI. Given a task to do, hearing, or reading description words related to a specific aspect of value, reproducible brain activity should be possible.

Also, if each aspect of value were presented to a person, some would show more activity than others. Which aspects of value showed more activity could likely be postulated from an inter-personal tools and weapons survey and/or asking earliest memories.

2) A survey could be used to rate the use of interpersonal tools and weapons, friends, or couples could use to rate each other. If the results of my own experiment are reproducible, what they say they would not like to be called, "heartless, stupid, lazy, or weak," should predict the way they rate other people, especially in what their best attribute was. For qualities, the aspects of value could be used, or "justice, Temperance (patience/balance), Knowledge/Wisdom, Humanity, Courage, Virtue, Transcendence(Optimism/vision)" In my study I wish I would have asked them to rate them in order instead of just picking their best quality.

3) A game could be played within a group, a scenario acted out, or a story told, and then people could be asked to recall the event. What details each person remembers or forgets likely will be correlated to their earliest memories, or an inter-personal tools and weapons. Also the story will likely be told using descriptive words associated with their preferred emotional lens.

4) The earliest memories and how someone approached a problem seem to have a very consistent correlation. Simulating a problem that could be solved equally seven

different ways would probably be difficult, but which career or hobbies they have chosen should work. Already I have seen for instance that surprise lens promotes a career in medicine or psychology, and sadness lens promotes a career in engineering or construction.

5) Asked earliest memories and then asked to rate a list of what triggers them and what makes them excited, there should be a correlation. For example, a person with happiness as an early memory would be more sensitive to rejection. Because there would likely be bias in what someone wants to identify that triggers them, a friend or partner could also answer.

6) In some therapy modality like sand-play therapy, three sand boxes could be there with labels, "How other people see us," "How we want to see ourselves," and "What feels like part of us but we don't like to show anybody." This would represent the persona, the ego, and the shadow, and would be consistent with their earliest memories, and the words they use to describe things now.

7) Have a patient rate their order of preference for each tool and weapon. Or label the top three ideal tools in other people's eyes, and top three for themselves. Label the top three most tabooed weapons in other people eyes and top three for themselves. Label the three most easily rationalized weapons both in their own eyes and in others. These results should end up being consistent with childhood memories, factors in current struggles, and show consistent activity on fMRI.

8) Write 21 different scenarios, one for each interpersonal tool where it is the optimal tool, but have the scenario vague enough that it's not self-evident what the appropriate tool is. Have a person respond which tool they would try first in that situation, what tool they would try second, and which weapon they would use if they needed to. These results should end up being consistent with childhood memories, factors in current struggles, and show consistent activity on fMRI.

9) In psycho-pharmacology there are a few tricks to knowing which medication will work best, for example the difference between depression where someone eats more and atypical depression where someone eats less determines the difference in the effectiveness of an SSRI versus an SNRI. In most other situations, there are general approaches for

diagnosis like bi-polar or schizophrenia, but it is usually a matter or trying different medications until one works, which takes months for each medication change to show cost versus benefit. Whenever a neuro-circuit is used, growth hormone is secreted, and that pathway is strengthened or widened. If the twenty-one tools and weapons are fundamentally connected to specific neuro-pathways, then clinical manifestations of psycho-pathologies could be cross-talk or counter currents at cross points where two pathways have widened to the point where they overlap electrically. This would create twenty-one different possible types of temporal lobe epilepsy. Being that neither serotonin, dopamine, or norepinephrine are intrinsically "happy hormones," it could be that the functionality of psychotropic medications is direct de-emphasis of areas of widened pathways, or indirect de-emphasis of widened pathways by emphasis in a complimentary part of the brain. Correlating a survey and/or assessment of which interpersonal weapons are most and least tabooed to which medication ends up actually working, could help predict which medication would work before just trying them.

9780692134931